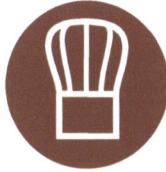

Table of Contents

Introduction

My name is Zachari Breeding, AKA Mr. Cook-It. I am a professional chef and registered dietitian (RD).

I earned a Bachelor of Science in Culinary Arts from The Restaurant School at Walnut Hill College in 2006 and a Masters of Science degree in Clinical Nutrition at New York University in 2015. In order to obtain the RD credential, I completed my dietetic internship at New York University Langone Medical Center (NY, NY) and Stamford Hospital (Stamford, CT). I have studied culinary arts and nutrition in France, England, and Italy, learning about various styles of food preparation, wine, and the influence of various cultures on cuisine.

Professionally, I own and operate a catering and personal nutrition business since 2007. I developed my unique presence in nutrition by working in clinical and community settings providing Medical Nutrition Therapy and Nutrition Counseling in the South Bronx and Brooklyn, New York. I am the owner and site manager for **the-sage.org**, a food and nutrition website.

My approach to nutrition therapy and counseling is based around the patient, where I provide an integrative approach using current evidence-based research, outcome development, and personal recipe modifications.

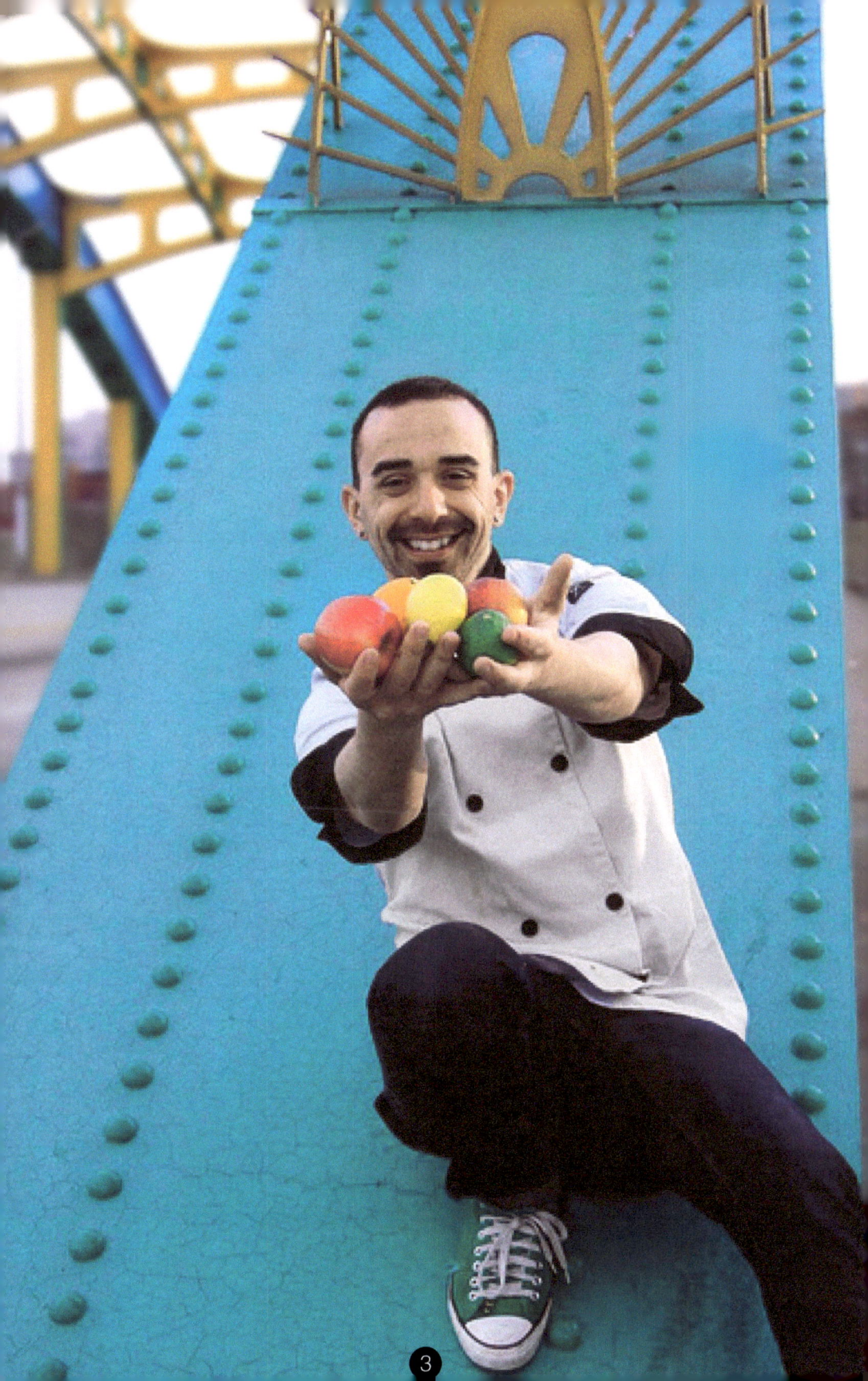

Focus

There is an old adage I learned as a child: "It's as simple as a slice of bread." This saying is the basis of this plan. Because let's face it - Diets are hard.

If you ever wondered why it is so easy to start any other popular or "fad" diet and JUST as easy to come off, it's because they are just that, a fad. Like any pop group boy band from the late 90's, these things come and go. But your health is forever.

So what do you do?

When you start a "diet," motivation is high, dedication is high, and excitement is built by the anticipation of results. After a few weeks, the excitement becomes anxiety, the motivation begins to wear, and dedication starts to deteriorate. The concept of starting something new is now routine, and weight loss may be gradual. Once the routine is underway, you start to get bored. Then, you get anxious from not getting faster results. We always want things to happen fast, don't we? If results are achieved, most of the time that is when the diet is discontinued. If not, it is an inevitable occurrence. After all, the "diet" was made to achieve a goal; once the goal is achieved, you think... "I can eat what I want, now."

Why does weight loss have to equal total restriction of the foods you enjoy? What is wrong with rapid weight loss? How do you deal with the humdrum of routine dietary changes? Most importantly, where do the not-so-healthy foods you enjoy fit into a healthy lifestyle?

Moderation

The key to a lifestyle change is moderation, not complete elimination of all your favorite "unhealthy foods". This is a cliché saying that has been popping up everywhere in the media. Here are some tips about what IS and what IS NOT considered moderation:

• It *IS* maintaining a balanced healthful eating regimen

• It *IS* including treats and "unhealthy" foods on occasion

• It *IS NOT* dedicating several meals a week to "unhealthy foods."

• It *IS NOT* excusing the entire day to bad eating habits because one meal went less than expected.

• It *IS NOT* eating multiple servings of your favorite "treats" at one sitting.

• It *IS* something you can do.

Talking about moderation leaves it up to the individual to decide what is moderate. There is some merit to this method and mantra because humans can also be quite obsessive – there are many people doing an exclusion diet (low carb, no grains, no gluten, no added sugars, etc.). These people seem to have a lot of anxiety about food in general, especially when it comes to how much to eat. No one should stress about food, that's why "diets" don't typically work in the long-term. Whole foods are rich in good nutrition, leaving room for that brownie, bag of chips, or soda you may crave every now and then. I would recommend limiting these foods to about 3x per week, which fits right under the manta of "moderation." This ensures that you lead a healthy, balanced diet without complete restriction of any one food - processed or not.

Unhealthy Weight Loss Short Cuts

Rapid weight loss seems very attractive, let's be real. There are gallon-sized drinks at the local pharmacy to "LOSE 20 POUNDS IN 2 WEEKS," shakes and meal substitution bars to promote rapid weight loss, even pills that use a variety of mechanisms to drop the pounds. In order to understand why THIS PLAN WILL WORK, we need to understand why these other ones do not.

WEIGHT LOSS IN A JUG

Simply put, these juices are nothing more than a sweetened flavored beverage with a multivitamin mixed in (and sometimes a lot of caffeine). The large amount of sugar in these beverages attracts the fluid within your body's cells. Once this is bound together, you urinate it out (if you have ever tried one of these drinks you know you are constantly using the restroom).

Not only are you constantly urinating the fluid from your cells (causing presumed "weight loss"), but you are reducing the amount of calories you eat per day by so much that your body begins to go into starvation mode. You are not consuming enough protein or fat that your body needs to run, so your body begins to run on the quickly-broken-down processed sugars from the drinks. Whenever you cut calories, no matter how unhealthfully, you will lose weight. That is a fact. However, once these drinks are discontinued, the joy of the temporary weight loss is short lived as the weight quickly returns along with the fluid within your cells.

These drinks also have a gamut of side effects including:
• Diarrhea
• Nausea
• Gas and Bloating
• Liver and Kidney Issues
• Irritability, Rapid Heart Rate

...And so many more. These side effects depend on the ingredient list, and most people do not research the ingredients on these products. It is also important to know that these products are considered dietary supplements, which are not regulated or evaluated by the Food and Drug Administration (FDA). At this time, there are no concrete current standards on said products. This is the reason these products are on the market, preying on those who are looking for a quick fix.

SHAKE IT OFF

The idea behind the many weight loss shakes of the world (including the ones you prepare at home) is to replace a meal as well as contain sugar and protein.

Weight loss shakes are high calorie, high protein beverages used to make the person "skip" a meal, allowing them to consume overall less calories a day. If a weight loss drink contains about 350 calories, this can be about half the amount a person would normally consume with a sandwich and a bag of chips. The sugar in these drinks can come from fruit or fruit juice (think homemade ones), processed sugar, honey, agave... you name it. Your blood sugar is then spiked super high, which over time can lead to bigger health issues. The point is, these carbohydrates help make the claim that this is a meal replacement, since the amount is usually pretty high. In drinking a shake, you fill your body with a lot of sugar and protein- but lacking the fiber, nutrients, and natural essence of food that comes from eating a balanced meal. Plus – could you do this for life?

The problem is that these drinks do not have much sustenance. Calorically, they should replace a meal to promote weight loss, but drinking a can of thickened liquid does not keep you feeling full for very long. You may even eat something with a shake, which defeats the purpose of reducing total caloric intake in an effort to lose weight. This person is better off eating a balanced, good tasting, healthy meal.

SWALLOW FOR "GOOD HEALTH"

With the variety of over the counter pills on the market to promote weight loss, it is so easy to get mixed up in the confusion, pick one, and eat whatever you want. Some people even think that, along with a diet, weight loss drugs are beneficial in hastening the effects. In reality, these drugs are all very different from one another and should be treated as such.

Orlistat: Orlistat-containing drugs are the first weight loss drugs endorsed by the Food and Drug Administration. The ingredient orlistat prevents fat from absorbing into the bloodstream from within the stomach. In doing so, the fat resumes transit through the gastrointestinal tract, leaving through the rectum. This can result in anal leakage and loss of control of stool. There are also concerns regarding the absorption of fat-soluble vitamins – weight loss at the price of a vitamin deficiency? No thanks. However, orlistat is clinically proven to promote weight loss by simply reducing the amount of fat digested.

Appetite Suppressants: Through a variety of ingredients and mechanisms, these drugs do just that: suppress one's appetite. Alone, these are not so bad. However, when combined with a fat burner, stimulant, or other type of not-so-great drug, the potential consequences seem to outweigh the potential benefits. Though the idea of eating less by suppressing the appetite seems attractive, it is important to understand why the appetite is high to begin with. Prolonged eating of large amounts of food results in continued release of hormones that call for hunger, despite the lack of needing energy from food. Over time with a diet of moderation, these hormones will subside and your appetite will resume to a more natural pace. Additionally, consuming foods adequate in nutrients and fiber will subside the appetite from returning quickly.

"Fat Burners": These drugs have been on the market for the longest period of time. Even though they no longer contain ephedra (a commonly used weight loss ingredient that has since been deemed dangerous and has been discontinued), the other ingredients may result in rapid heart rate, heart attack, and stroke. They may suppress hunger and in eating less, your body begins to drop weight. The weight loss is, for the most part, lean muscle, since protein is the next source of energy during times of increased metabolism. Some fat is lost, but losing fat is not as easy as popping a pill.

Any and all of these drugs have varying side effects based on the ingredients listed. Some of these ingredients have interactions with medications you may already be taking and cause severe interactions. Although it is best to avoid such drugs when beginning a weight loss regime, consult with a physician first before taking any weight loss medication.

Don't be fooled by mystery ingredients or popularized promotions. If you do not understand the items in the ingredients statement, you are better off not taking it. Chances are if you researched all of the ingredients, you would not want to take it anyway. Even though your favorite TV-doctor program endorses a product or a physician is shown on the label, these products are not regulated by the Food and Drug Administration and lack definitive studies proving their safety and efficacy.

Any drink, shake, bar, or pill you take may have desired results. They also may carry potential significant health consequences and drug interactions. If the risk seems worth the potential benefit it is up to you. Most people who start a weight loss regime this way not only do not continue for a lifetime, and most regain the weight back.

This plan for a long lasting lifestyle change has been created with all of this in mind... with YOU in mind. Because losing weight can be tough, frustrating, and disappointing. And there is no easy way out. As we go through this process together, I will show you how to start eating the right way and with foods YOU enjoy. This way, weight loss will be gradual, healthy, and lifelong. It can be "as simple as a slice of bread."

A Slice of Information

"Carbs are not the enemy."

The idea behind this plan is to reduce the amount of carbohydrates you eat every day. Of course, there are carbohydrates in many other foods. The purpose of this plan, however, is to focus on carbohydrates from starches – grains, starchy vegetables, and legumes (beans, etc.) It is important to know that CARBS ARE NOT THE ENEMY, but they can contribute to weight gain when eaten in excess (which they usually are).

Studies show that the biggest culprit in weight gain from fat is from carbohydrates, especially refined and processed ones from grains. The sugars in these foods break down quickly and when they cannot be used for energy, turn into fat in your body. Consuming your slices as WHOLE GRAINS is the best choice here, and limiting them is paramount. Complete restriction of carbohydrates will lead to drowsiness and fatigue, loss of muscle function, and impaired organ and brain function.

You may enjoy the foods you choose to be your slices any way you wish, but recommendations for selected meals are below. It is REQUIRED that you eat the same amount of slices per meal, with extras being left for snacks, if applicable.

For instance, if you are allotted 10 slices, the following daily meal plan should be followed:

Breakfast (3), Snack #1 (1/2), Lunch (3), Dinner (3), Snack #2 (1/2)

Recipes follow later in the booklet. The basic concept of this plan is to continue consuming carbohydrates and prepare your body to metabolize them efficiently, which means eating the same amount each day. Your metabolism will be kept high by enjoying two snacks per day- one between breakfast and lunch, the other at night after dinner. The amount of Slices you are allotted depends on age, gender, height, weight, and physical activity level. This plan is not recommended for those under the age of 18. Please consult a pediatrician or pediatric dietitian for weight loss recommendations.

Because you do not need to have grains sitting in your system at night, nighttime snacks should include different foods than your daytime snack. Snack suggestions follow later in this booklet.

Confused? At the end of this booklet is contact information for you to ask any question along the way, get additional recipes, and get the help you need. The best part about this plan is knowing you are not alone- that a professional registered dietitian and chef is only a few keystrokes away from peace of mind.

Now, let's look at what constitutes "a slice."

What is a Slice?

Grains & Pastas

Breakfast	Lunch	Dinner	Snacks
¼ bagel	1 slice bread	1/3 cup pasta	8 animal crackers
1 biscuit	½ cup couscous	1/3 cup barley	6 regular crackers
½ english muffin	¼ piece naan bread	½ cup grits	3 graham crackers
One 4" pancake/ waffle	½ hot dog bun	1/3 cup polenta	20 oyster crackers
½ cup breakfast cereal	½ hamburger bun	1/3 cup rice	3 cups popcorn
¼ cup granola or muesli	½ 6" piece pita bread	1/3 cup stuffing	¾ oz pretzels
1 slice bread/ toast	1- 6" tortilla: flour/corn	One 1" cube cornbread	2 rice cakes
½ cup oats	1/3- 10" tortilla	2 taco shells	¾ oz snack chips
½ cup fruit juice	1/3 cup quinoa	1/3 cup risotto	¾ oz tortilla chips

Remember to select whole grains when possible

ONE SLICE = 15 GRAMS CARBOHYDRATE

Vegetables & Beans

- ½ cup potato, cooked
- ½ cup parsnips
- 1 cup winter squash
  - butternut
  - spaghetti
  - acorn
- ½ cup beans, any kind
- ½ cup peas
- 1/3 cup plantains
- ½ cup yam/sweet potato
- 1/3 cup baked beans
- ½ cup corn (1/2 cob)
- 1 cup pumpkin
- 1 cup mixed vegetables
- ½ cup lentils

Prepared Foods

- ½ cup casserole with noodles or rice
- 1/8 (1 slice) pizza - thin/regular crust (varies)
- 1 cup canned soup
- ½ cup ramen noodles
- ½ pot pie
- 1 cup stew with pasta/rice
- 1/3 microwavable pocket sandwich
- ½ cup potato salad
- 1/3 of a 5 oz burrito
- 1/3 of a small fast food French fries
- 1/3 of a 6" submarine sandwich
- 1 egg roll
- 4 oz hummus

Free Foods

The following foods are considered "free" and can be consumed unlimited.

This includes fresh or cooked fruits (fruit juice or canned fruits in syrup excluded), and fresh or cooked non-starchy vegetables (excluded from the list above).

How many Slices?

Men Ages 18 — 50 *

Physical Activity Level Not Included **

height → / weight →

height \ weight	120	130	140	150	160	170	180	190	200	220	240	260	280	300
6'8"						14	14	14	14	14	13	14	14	15
6'6"					14	14	14	14	14	13	13	14	14	14
6'4"				14	14	14	14	14	13	13	13	14	14	14
6'2"			14	14	14	14	14	13	13	13	13	14	14	14
6'		13	13	14	14	14	13	13	13	13	13	14	14	14
5'10"		12	12	13	13	12	12	13	13	13	13	14	13	13
5'8"		12	12	12	12	11	11	12	12	12	13	13	13	13
5'6"	10	10	11	11	10	10	10	11	12	12	13	13	13	13
5'4"	10	10	10	10	10	10	11	11	12	12	12	13	13	13
5'2"	9	9	10	10	10	11	11	11	11	12	12	12	13	13
5'	9	8	9	10	10	11	11	11	11	12	12	12	13	13
4'10"	9	9	9	8	8	8	8	9	9	9	10	10	10	10
4'8"	8	8	7	7	7	8	8	8	9	9	9	10	10	10
4'6"	8	7	7	7	7	7	8	8	8	9	9	9	10	10

*For Men Ages 50+, subtract 1 slice daily.

14

Women Ages 18 — 50 *

Physical Activity Level Not Included **

height \ weight	120	130	140	150	160	170	180	190	200	220	240	260	280	300
6'8"						12	12	12	12	12	11	12	12	13
6'6"					12	12	12	12	12	11	11	12	12	12
6'4"				12	12	12	12	12	11	11	11	12	12	12
6'2"			12	12	12	12	12	11	11	11	11	12	12	12
6'		11	12	11	11	12	11	11	10	11	11	12	12	12
5'10"		10	11	10	10	10	10	10	9	11	11	12	12	12
5'8"		8	10	9	10	9	9	9	10	10	11	11	11	11
5'6"	8	8	9	8	10	8	8	9	10	10	11	11	11	11
5'4"	8	8	8	8	10	8	9	9	10	10	10	10	11	11
5'2"	8	7	8	8	8	8	9	9	9	10	10	10	11	11
5'	8	7	8	8	6	8	8	9	9	10	10	10	11	11
4'10"	7	7	7	6	6	6	6	7	7	7	8	8	8	8
4'8"	6	6	7	5	6	6	6	6	7	7	7	8	8	8
4'6"	6	5	5	5	5	6	6	6	6	7	7	7	8	8

*For Women Ages 50+, subtract 1 slice daily.

** Physical Activity Levels:

Light (75-125 minutes per week): add 1 slice daily

Moderate (125-200 minutes per week): add 2 slices daily

Heavy (over 200 minutes per week): add 3 slices daily

The Plan

So now, you should have an idea on how many "Slices" you are allotted per day. This counts for carbohydrate intake, only. It also includes mixed meals with starches, legumes (lentils and beans), and starchy vegetables (corn, potatoes, peas, etc.).

But what about the other food groups? If carbohydrates aren't the enemy (which they are certainly not), then what about meat, dairy, fruits, and non-starchy vegetables? The focus on this plan is to REDUCE the amount of carbohydrates, but that does not mean you can have your cheese, steak, cake, and eat it too. For protein and dairy foods, keep cheese/meat/meat-substitute portions no bigger than a deck of cards (4 oz.) per meal and dairy (yogurt, milk) no more than 6 oz. per meal (choose Low Fat or Fat Free). Try not to exceed eggs 5 times per week. If you combine cheese with meat/meat-substitutes, do not exceed the 4 oz. rule.

The Sweet Tooth

You'll notice I did not include cakes and sweets as part of the "Slices." This is because, even though these foods are obviously carbohydrates, they are not part of a healthy diet. More specifically, it would not be wise to eat 3 "Slices" worth of chocolate for lunch and no other carbohydrate, right?

Keep it realistic. Keep your sweets each day **under 200 calories**. You will need to check the Nutrition Facts Label for calorie information, since these numbers vary by product. Baking on your own is a great idea, but tends to lead to higher consumption (since it is always existent in your home) and lack of nutritional information. My advice is to pick-up a dessert while you are out on days you think you might want something sweet and keep fruits in your home at all times to satisfy the craving. Some suggestions are:

• Dark Chocolate pieces (less milk means less fat) – at least 72% cocoa

• Slow-Churned Ice Cream (naturally less fat)

• Honey Roasted Peanuts or Cocoa/Cinnamon – Dusted Almonds

• Fruit Sorbet

• Frozen Yogurt Pops

• Italian Ice

• Meringue Cookies

• Skinny Cow® products (or dessert products made with skim milk

As for the other food groups, the best example to review is the most updated version of the healthy eating model from the Dietary Guidelines for Americans by the USDA (United States Department of Agriculture) based on a 9" plate. This is called MyPlate:

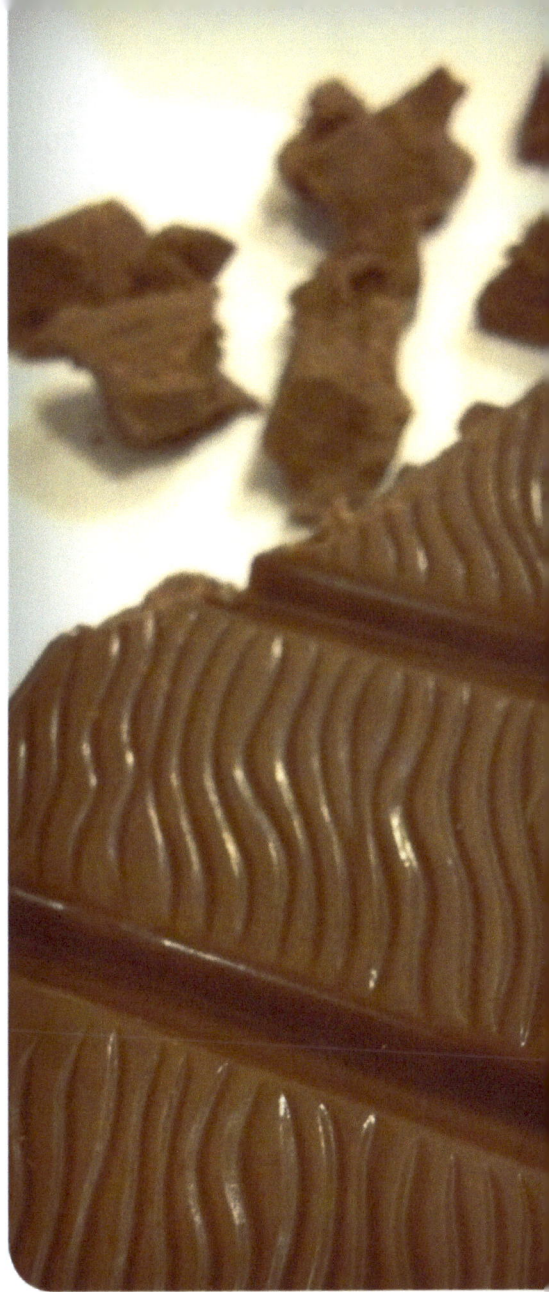

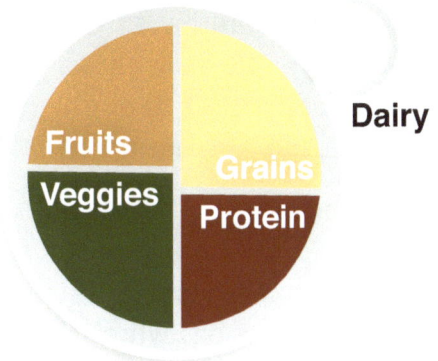

Every meal should look like this plate! If half of your plate is all fruit or all vegetables, do not worry, because this is just fine! Start to Think Healthier & Consider the following:

Group	Choose LESS often	Choose MORE often
Carbohydrates	White bread, rice, tortillas, pasta	Whole grain/whole wheat bread, tortilla, pita, pasta, brown rice
	Sugar coated cereal	Oatmeal, granola, shredded wheat
	Dessert foods, sweets	Fresh fruit
Juices	Fruit juices and smoothies	Make your own in a blender (keep the fiber!)
Dairy	Full fat cheese and milk	Nonfat or 1% milk, cheese, yogurt, cottage cheese
Protein	Red meat: steak, hamburger	Chicken breast, turkey, beans, eggs, pork, tofu, venison
Fats	Butter, mayonnaise, lard	Nuts, avocado, coconut, olive oil
Seafood	Shellfish (higher in cholesterol)	Fish: salmon, haddock, cod, halibut, tuna
Drinks	Soda, fruit juice, sugary drinks	Water, diet soda, coffee/tea + artificial sweetener
Fast Food	Fried/breaded foods, soft drinks	Grilled foods, fresh fruit, salads, water
Cooking Methods	Frying, deep-frying with: butter, crisco, lard	Steaming, baking, blanching, grilling, sautéing with: olive, sesame, canola, soybean, vegetable oil

Free Foods:
All fresh fruits and non-starchy vegetables are considered "free" and can be eaten throughout the day with meals and as snacks. Limit fruit juices without pulp (fiber) since these juices are usually high in sugar (carbohydrates) and are therefore reduced in nutritional value.

Alcohol:
Limit 2 drinks per day for men and 1 per day for women. A drink constitutes the following: (1) 12 oz. beer, 1 oz. (a shot) liquor, and 5 oz. wine (red or white).

Meal Examples

Day	Breakfast	AM Snack	Lunch	Dinner	PM Snack
Mon	6 oz. yogurt ½ c. granola ½ c. berries	Carrot sticks, 2 oz. hummus	1/2 Veggie Burrito*	Garden lasagna*, romaine salad	2 oz. low fat cheese, grapes
Tue	1 c. skim milk, ½ c. shredded wheat, 1 apple	celery sticks, peanut butter, 2 oz. raisins	1 pita, 2 TB tzatziki*, 2 c. spinach salad	Halibut + strawberry salsa* (1 cup), quinoa, green salad	6 oz. yogurt, roasted almonds
Wed	2 eggs scrambled, ½ c. cooked kale, 1 english muffin, 1 oz. cheese	½ pita, 2 TB salsa, 1 TB shredded cheese	1 portion of beet potato walnut salad*, oyster crackers	Chicken with apple salsa*, 2/3 c. brown rice, steamed asparagus	1 apple, Walnuts or 1 TB peanut butter
Thu	¼ bagel with 2 TB peanut butter 1 banana, 6 oz. yogurt	1.5 cups popcorn	1 can tuna fish + 1 TB mayo + 2 slices wheat bread, celery sticks	2/3 cup pasta, ½ cup tomato sauce, romaine & spinach salad	3 crackers, 1 large or 3 small slices low fat sharp cheddar cheese
Fri	½ c. oatmeal + 1 TB peanut butter 1 apple	Animal crackers, 6 oz. yogurt	Mixed green salad, fruit, 2 oz. low fat cheese	2 pc. veggie pizza*, baked honey chipotle wings*	Almonds, fruit, ¾ oz. pretzels
Sat	2 eggs (hard boiled), ½ c. black beans, 2 TB salsa, 1 sm. Tortilla, ½ c. raw spinach	2 rice cakes, 1 TB peanut butter ½ apple	1 slice garlic toast, ratatouille*, 2 TB shredded mozzarella cheese	Lamb +mango chutney*, 1 portion papas bravas*, sautéed green beans	½ cup pumpkin smoothie*, ¼ cup almonds
Sun	1 pancake + 1 TB syrup + 1 pear, 1 cup lowfat milk	¾ oz baked tortilla chips, ½ c. salsa	Pulled chicken sandwich*, baby carrots	Asian lettuce wraps*, ½ cup brown rice	¾ oz pretzels, 1 TB peanut butter

* See Recipe

Recipes

Ribollita

ONE SERVING = 2 SLICES ON THE SLICE PLAN

Preparation Time: approximately 25 minutes
Cooking Time: 60 minutes
Serving Size: approximately 2 cups (Makes 4)

INGREDIENTS

1/4 cup	Olive oil
3 TB	Garlic, chopped
2- 15.5 oz cans	Great Northern beans
4 oz	Pancetta, diced (optional)
2	Onions, yellow, diced
4	Carrots, diced small
4	Celery, diced small
1/4 tsp	Crushed red pepper flakes
1- 28 oz can	San Marzano Tomatoes (whole canned tomatoes will do also)
6 cups	Chicken or Vegetable stock, low sodium
1 bunch	Kale, chopped rough
1 cup	Basil, chopped rough
2 TB	Thyme, minced
4 cups	Sourdough bread, stale/hard in 2" cubes
To Taste	Kosher Salt and Black Pepper
2 tsp	Nutmeg
1 TB	Granulated sugar
1/2 cup	Parmesan cheese, grated

DIRECTIONS

Heat oil in large pot. Sauté garlic until aromatic over medium—high heat.

Add onions and sauté until onions become slightly translucent. Add carrots, celery, and red pepper flakes and cook 10 minutes. Add tomatoes and chicken stock; stir and cover, allow to simmer for 20 minutes at medium—low heat.

Add kale and basil and toss until all of the kale is submerged. Stir in the beans; continue cooking over medium heat for about 20 minutes uncovered. Add the stale bread cubes to the pot and stir around once lightly to prevent breaking up the bread. Turn off heat, cover, and let sit for 10 minutes.

Turn-out & Storage:
Top with Parmesan cheese.

May be stored under refrigeration without bread for 3 days - add bread upon reheating. Otherwise, the bread will absorb too much of the broth!

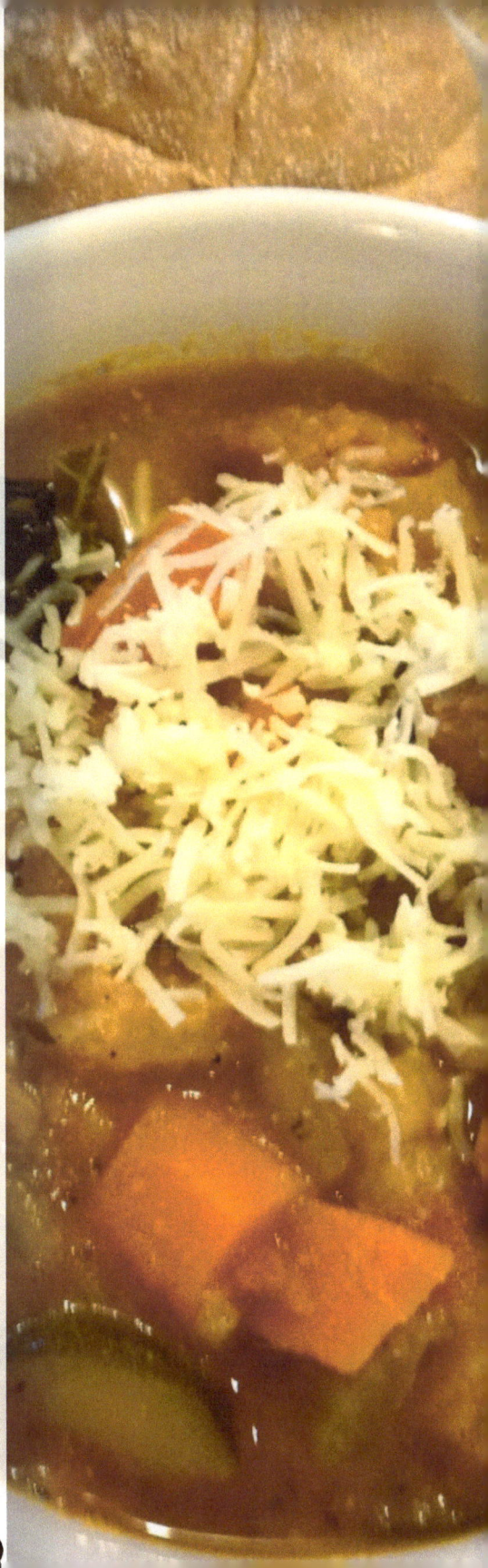

Papas Bravas

ONE SERVING = 1 SLICE ON THE SLICE PLAN

Preparation Time: approximately 10 minutes
Cooking Time: 25 minutes
Serving Size: ½ cup (Makes 6)

INGREDIENTS

5......................... potatoes, redskin, large
1 cup.................. vegetable oil
1 TB.................... garlic, minced
8 oz .... tomato sauce, canned, no-salt added
2 tsp .... Dijon mustard
1/8 tsp................ hot sauce
½ tsp.................. sugar
To Taste .... salt

DIRECTIONS

Heat oil in skillet. Cut potatoes into medium sized wedges, 8 per potato. Add to oil and fry, tossing occasionally to brown all sides, until al dente. Drain oil, reserving 1 TB. Sprinkle potatoes with salt.

Meanwhile, sauté garlic in reserved oil. Add tomato sauce, mustard, sugar, and hot sauce. Season with salt. Simmer 5 minutes.

Turn-out & Storage:
Pour sauce over potatoes and serve hot. Garnish with ripped fresh parsley leaves.

May be stored under refrigeration for up to 3 days.

Black Bean & Vegetable Enchilada Casserole

ONE SERVING = 1 SLICE ON THE SLICE PLAN

Preparation Time: approximately 15-20 minutes
Cooking Time: 30-45 minutes
Serving Size: 3x3" square piece (Makes 12)

INGREDIENTS

2 TB	olive oil
1	red onion, diced
2 TB	garlic, chopped
1/2 lb.	mushrooms, sliced thick
2	red bell peppers, diced
1	zucchini, medium, medium diced
1 ½ cups	brown rice, prepared (per directions on label)
4 oz	corn, frozen (thawed)
4 oz	spinach, baby (fresh)
15.5 oz	NSA* fired roasted tomatoes, diced
1 TB	cumin
2 tsp	coriander
1 TB	chili powder
2 tsp	oregano, dried (or 1 TB freshly minced)
2 tsp	garlic powder
2 tsp	onion powder
1 tsp	salt
2 tsp	sugar, raw granules
2	green chilies, sliced
2	jalapeños, diced (optional)
16 oz	black beans, rinsed (NSA* canned or dry prepared)
1 ½ cup	shredded cheese: cheddar or Monterey jack (part-skim)
6-9	corn tortillas, baked**
2	avocados, sliced

DIRECTIONS

Preheat oven to 350 degrees. Grease a 9x13" baking pan with cooking spray or dabbing a paper towel with olive oil.

Heat the fire roasted tomatoes in a saucepot over medium heat. Add cumin, coriander, chili powder, oregano, and garlic/onion powders. Season with salt and raw sugar as directed or to taste. Set aside.

Meanwhile, heat olive oil in a large skillet or braiser/rondeau. Sauté onions and garlic until transluscent; add bell peppers and zucchini and cook until softened slightly. Add mushrooms, corn, and chili peppers and toss together, cooking until slightly soft as well. Set aside.

Layer three tortillas (broken into thirds) on the base of the baking pan. Layer with half of the vegetable mixture. Top with ¾ cup prepared rice followed by half of the beans then a third of the tomato sauce. Repeat again: tortillas, vegetable mixture, rice, beans, and sauce. Top with a third layer of tortilla pieces then the remainder of the sauce followed by jalapeño slices. Top with shredded cheese***. Cover and bake 30-40 minutes until internal temperature of 150 degrees is reached.

Turn-out & Storage: Serve immediately; garnish with avocado slices & cilantro sprig. Can be stored under refrigeration for up to 3 days.

*NSA: no salt added

**You can bake tortillas by placing them single layered on a baking sheet in the oven at 300 degrees for about 5-7 minutes. This will dry them out enough so they do not get mushy in the casserole baking process; the goal is to have them provide texture to this dish. Monitor their progress frequently after 5 minutes to prevent burning.

***You may split the cheese into 2 portions, adding a layer of cheese after the first layer of ingredients is placed in the baking pan, leaving the second portion for topping.

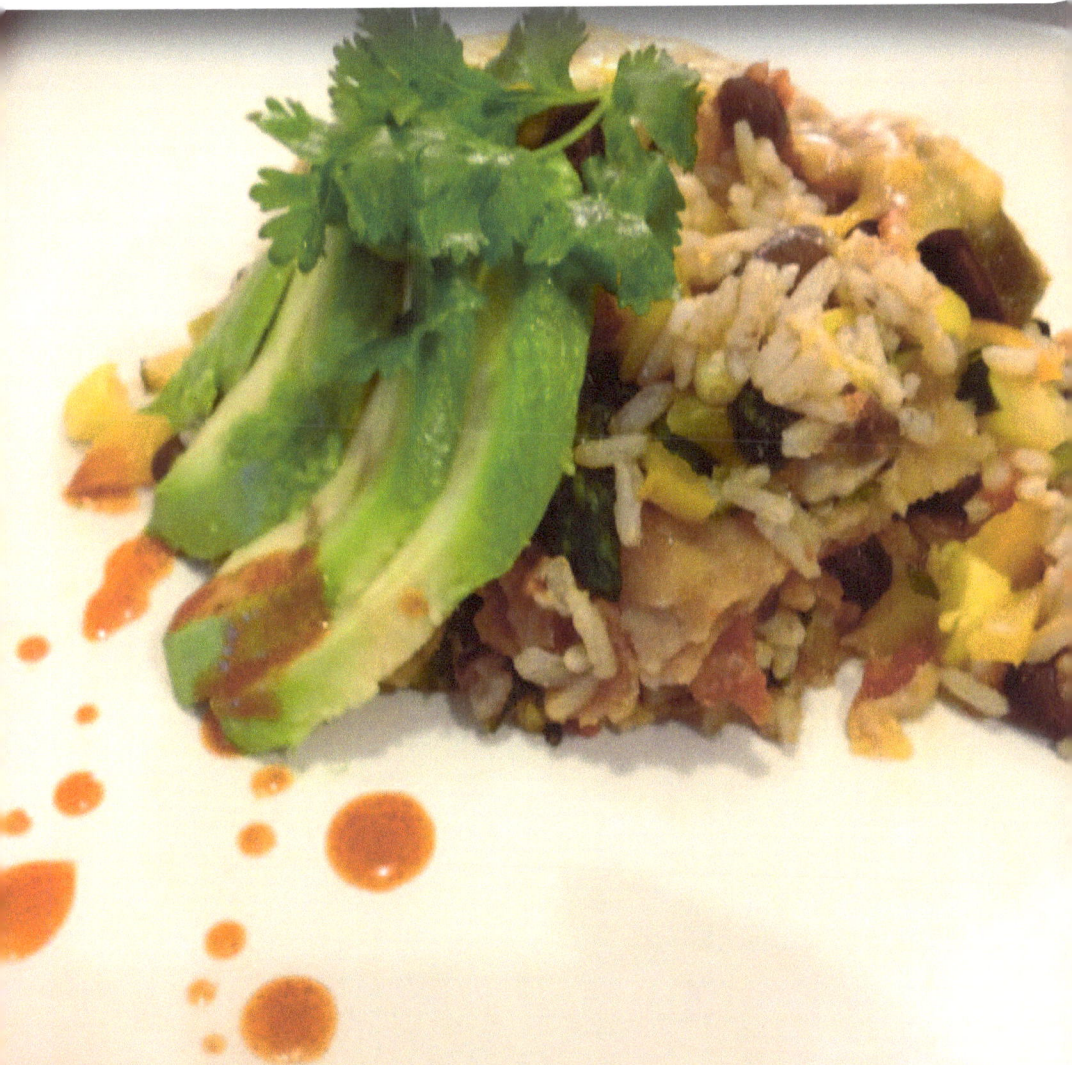

Spicy Roasted Tofu

ONE SERVING = 0 SLICES ON THE SLICE PLAN

Preparation Time: approximately 25 minutes
Cooking Time: 15-20 minutes
Serving Size: approximately ½ cup (Makes 4)

INGREDIENTS

1 lb. .... extra firm tofu, pressed & diced ½" cubes
2 TB................... olive oil
2 TB................... garlic, minced
1 tsp. .... Cajun spice blend
½ tsp. .... cayenne pepper
pinch................. black pepper
1 TB................... sesame oil
1 TB................... soy sauce, low-sodium

DIRECTIONS

Preheat oven to 400 degrees.
Toss together ingredients and
allow to marinate 20 minutes.

Give the mixture another
toss and spread out on
non-greased baking sheet
in one layer. Bake 15-20
minutes, rotating often, so
all sides have caramelized
and are golden brown.

Turn-out & Storage: Enjoy
chilled over a salad or
served hot with saffron rice
and roasted vegetables!
Can be stored under
refrigeration for up to 2 days.

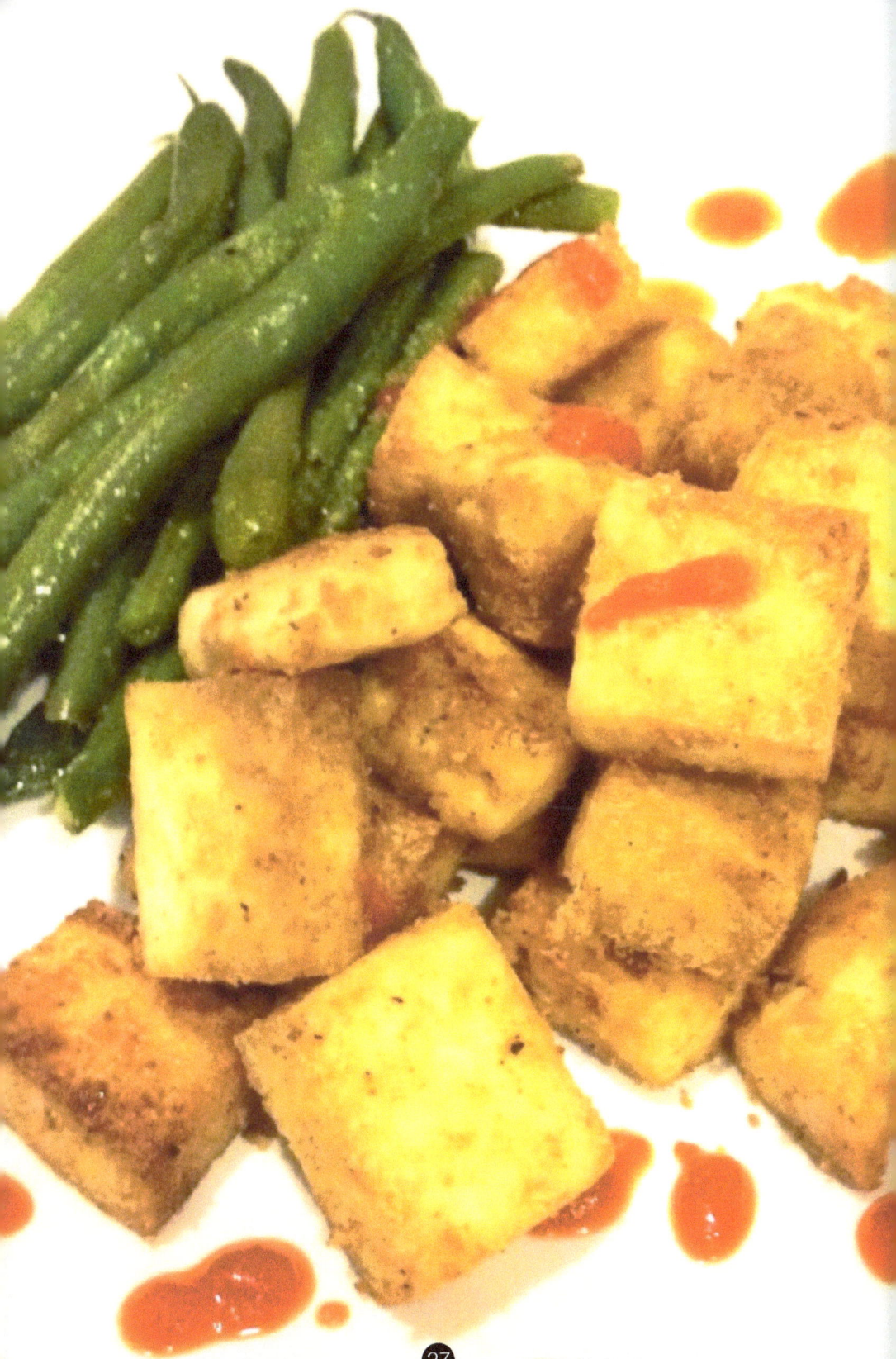

Roasted Vegetable Pizza

ONE SERVING = 3 SLICES ON THE SLICE PLAN

Preparation Time: approximately 20 minutes
Cooking Time: 50 minutes
Serving Size: 2 slices (Makes 8)

INGREDIENTS

½ .... doughball, pizza (prepared)
½ cup........... San Marzano Pizza Sauce (recipe follows)
½ .... zucchini, sliced ¼" thick
½ .... yellow squash, sliced ¼" thick
8 .... portabella mushrooms, sliced thick
¼ .... red onion, sliced thin
½ .... bell pepper, orange, julienned
¼ .... eggplant, quartered, sliced ½" thick
2 oz .... olive oil
1 TB............. Italian herb seasoning, dried*
2 tsp. .... garlic powder, dried
2 tsp. .... kosher salt
1 tsp. .... black pepper
8 oz .... mozzarella cheese, part-skim

San Marzano Pizza Sauce
1 TB .... olive oil
2 TB............. garlic, chopped
1 oz. .... red wine
28 oz........... San Marzano tomatoes
2 tsp. .... Italian herb seasoning, dried*
1 tsp. .... red pepper flakes
¾ tsp. .... kosher salt

DIRECTIONS

Preheat oven to 400 degrees. Grease a 9x13" baking pan with cooking spray or dabbing a paper towel with olive oil. Toss vegetables (zucchini, squash, eggplant, onion, bell pepper, mushrooms) in olive oil, Italian herb seasoning, garlic powder, kosher salt, and black pepper. Roast 10 minutes until halfway cooked and slightly browned on the bottom. Set aside to cool.

Preparing the sauce:
Meanwhile, sauté chopped garlic in olive oil 2-3 minutes, until softened. Deglaze the pan with red wine and allow to reduce for 1 minute. Add San Marzano tomatoes, Italian herb seasoning, red pepper flakes, and salt. Allow to simmer until thickened, about 20 minutes, stirring occasionally.
Roll out pizza dough and place on greased pizza pan.

Top with prepared pizza sauce. Bake at 400 degrees 8-10 minutes, until dough has risen slightly but remains very soft. Remove from oven and reduce heat to 350 degrees. Top with ¼ of mozzarella; top with veggie mix. Add remainder of mozzarella, and fresh herbs*. Bake 20-30 minutes until crust is golden brown and cheese has melted/caramelized or to desired doneness.

Turn-out & Storage: Allow to cool 5 minutes. Cut into 8 triangle slices or 9 square ones. Can be stored under refrigeration up to 3 days.

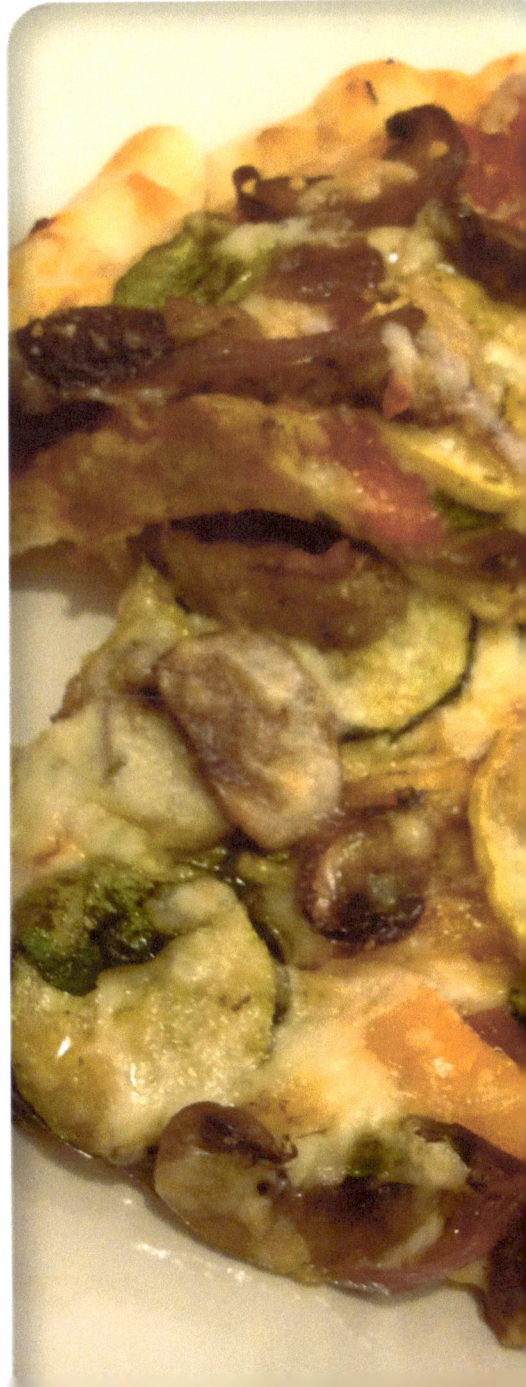

Tzatziki Sauce

ONE SERVING = 0 SLICES ON THE SLICE PLAN

Preparation Time: approximately 3-4 minutes
Cooking Time: N/a
Serving Size: approximately 2 TB (Makes about 4 cups)

INGREDIENTS

4 cups .... yogurt, plain
2 .... cucumbers, peeled and seeded, shredded
4 .... garlic cloves, smashed and minced
1 TB .... lemon juice
1 TB .... olive oil
¼ cup .... mint, chopped
To Taste .... salt and black pepper

DIRECTIONS

Strain yogurt in
cheesecloth over metal
colander for 3-4 hours.

Strain liquid from shredded
cucumber. Combine garlic,
salt, pepper, lemon juice,
olive oil. Add cucumber and
yogurt. Chill 1-2 hours.

Turn-out & Storage: This
can be stored for up to a
week under refrigeration.

Southwest Vegetarian Burritos

ONE SERVING = 5 SLICES ON THE SLICE PLAN

Preparation Time: approximately 15-20 minutes
Cooking Time: 15-20 minutes
Serving Size: 1 burrito (Makes 6)

<u>INGREDIENTS</u>

6	whole wheat tortillas, 10"
2 cups	fire-roasted tomatoes, canned, no salt added
2 cups	black beans, canned, no salt added*
2 cups	white beans, canned, no salt added, drained and rinsed*
3 TB	chipotle peppers in adobo sauce, chopped fine
1 cup	corn kernels, frozen and thawed**
2	red bell peppers, diced
1	red onion, diced
1 lb.	baby portabella or white mushrooms, cut into quarters
2 TB	garlic, chopped
2 cups	spinach (baby)
2 cups	brown rice, cooked
3	limes, juice of and zest of
½ bunch	cilantro, de-stemmed, washed, chopped
2 TB	cumin
1 TB	coriander
2 TB	chili powder
2 tsp/To Taste	cayenne pepper, ground
To Taste	salt
¼ cup	olive oil
1	avocado, sliced
1 cup	queso fresco, crumbled***

DIRECTIONS

Sauté 1 TB garlic in 1 TB olive oil until softened. Add cumin, coriander, chili powder, and cayenne – sauté 30 seconds, stirring constantly. Combine tomatoes, beans, chipotle, corn, and lime zest – add to pot. Allow to heat thoroughly (mixture will bubble). Season with salt and add ½ chopped cilantro. Reduce heat to low and set aside.

Meanwhile, heat 1 TB garlic and onion in remaining olive oil until softened. Add bell peppers and mushrooms and cook until al dente. Toss spinach into mixture last until wilted. Season with salt. Remove from heat, cover, and set aside.

Combine hot prepared brown rice with lime juice and ½ of the chopped cilantro. Season with salt. Set aside.

[Warm tortillas gently and only slightly (this can be done for about 15 seconds on high in the microwave or at 250 degrees for about 5 minutes in the oven) – overcooking these will result in gummy and rubbery tortillas.]

To fill: Lay tortilla flat and place 1/6 of rice mixture slightly to one side of middle. Top with 1/6 bean mixture followed by 1/6 vegetable mixture. Place avocado slices and crumbled cheese on top. Be careful not to overfill.

To wrap: Fold each side of tortilla inward at the same time, followed by the end with the least amount of space (remember you put the mixtures slightly to one side of the middle). Lift that side and make a big roll toward the opposite end, folding in after you have closed in the mixture. Fold the opposite end over and place folded sides down.

Turn-out & Storage: Cut in half and enjoy alone, alongside a mixed green salad with lime vinaigrette, or with baked tortilla chips!

Individual components of this recipe can be stored under refrigeration for up to 3 days.

*you may also use dried versions of the beans - just follow instructions on the product (canned is used here to reduce work load and prep time)

**canned corn is by far less nutritious than frozen corn, as it is cooked at a high temperature and canned with the vitamin-containing water that is drained out; quality is also reduced in the process

***you may use any low-fat cheese you prefer here, including Monterey Jack or Cheddar.

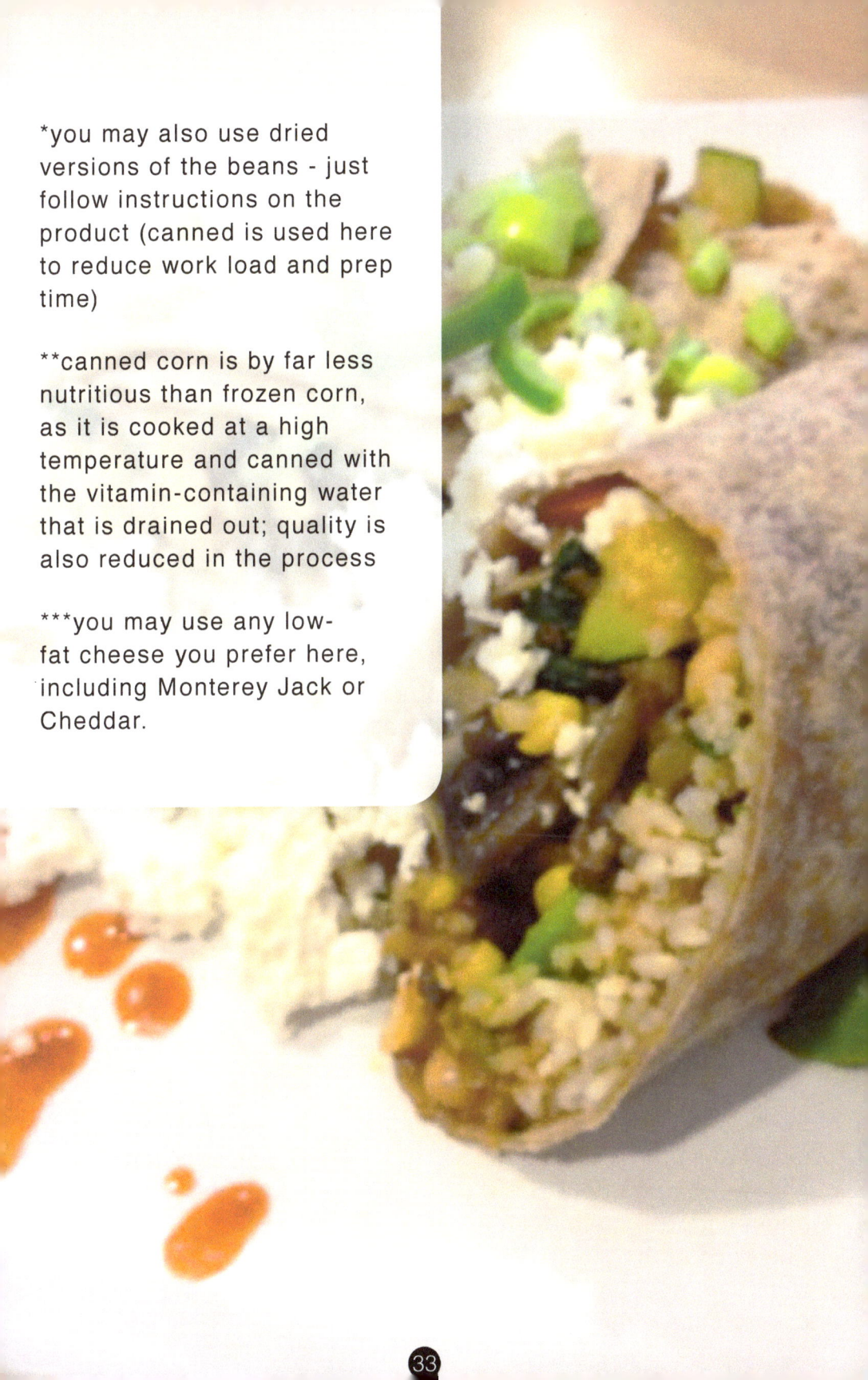

Tapenade Relish Stuffed Mushrooms

ONE SERVING = 0 SLICES ON THE SLICE PLAN

Preparation Time: approximately 10 minutes
Cooking Time: 10-15 minutes
Serving Size: 2 Mushrooms (Makes about 6)

INGREDIENTS

MUSHROOMS:

1 lb.	Portobello mushrooms, de-stemmed
4 TB....................	olive oil
1 ½ TB	Italian herb seasoning (dried)
2 tsp	salt
2 tsp	black pepper

RELISH:

8	olives, cured (kalamata, manzanilla, etc)* diced very small
½	large tomato, diced small
¼	small Vidalia onion, diced small
2 tsp	garlic, chopped
1 TB..................	basil, fresh, chopped
2 tsp	olive oil
1 TB..................	balsamic vinegar
2 tsp	salt
1 tsp	black pepper

DIRECTIONS

Preheat grill. Toss mushrooms in remaining ingredients and grill well on both sides, beginning with the cap side. The ends of the mushrooms will begin to soften and curl towards the center leaving black grilled marks indented on the top. Flip and continue grilling until mushrooms are al dente. (Try one to be sure!)

Meanwhile, combine all relish ingredients and allow to marinate at least 30 minutes. This is great to do while you are firing up the grill.

Remove mushrooms from grill and top with relish.

Turn-out & Storage:
This can be served alongside lemon-pepper seasoned grilled asparagus, couscous, grilled flatbread, roasted chickpeas, or grilled bell peppers.

Filling mixture can be stored under refrigeration for up to 5 days.

*These can be purchased commonly at the olive bar in your local grocery store! (Though some varieties come packaged.)

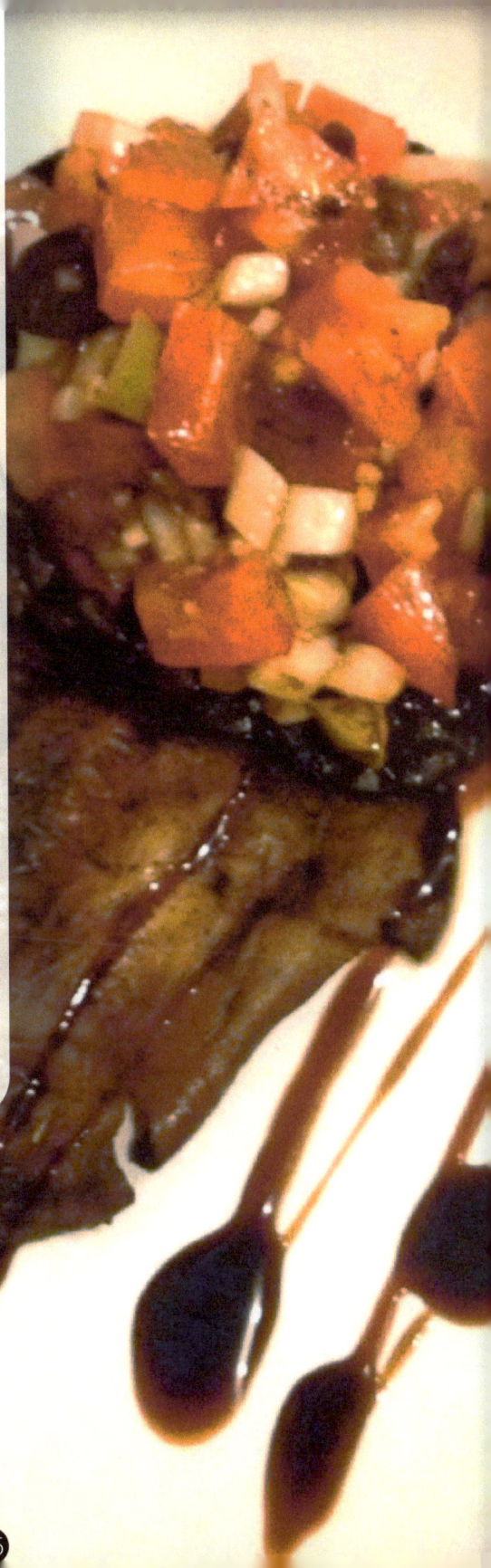

Ratatouille

ONE SERVING = 1 SLICE ON THE SLICE PLAN
(when served with bread)

Preparation Time: approximately 10 minutes
Cooking Time: 15-20 minutes
Serving Size: approximately 1 cup (Makes 5)

INGREDIENTS

¼ cup................. olive oil
2 TB.................... Garlic, minced
2 large .... Onions, yellow, small diced
6....................... Tomatoes, roma, large diced
2....................... Bell pepper, red, large diced
1....................... Bell pepper, green, large diced
1 large .... Eggplant, skin removed, diced into 1" cubes
4....................... Zucchini, medium/large, diced into 1" cubes
1- 15.5oz can ...... Cannellini beans, rinsed**
1 cup................. Parsley, chopped rough
½ cup................ Basil leaves, chopped rough
2 tsp .... Sugar, natural OR agave nectar
To Taste .... Kosher Salt and Black Pepper

DIRECTIONS

Heat oil in large skillet or braiser [rondeau]. Sauté garlic until aromatic over medium-high heat.

Add onions and sauté until onions become slightly translucent. Add bell peppers and toss occasionally for about 5 minutes. Add tomatoes, eggplant, and zucchini.

Cook until tomatoes have broken down, creating a sauce. Season with sugar, salt, and pepper. Add cannellini beans. Continue stirring occasionally until squashes are fork tender. Be careful not to stir too often as you could break the beans into pieces.

Toss in parsley and basil and cook an additional minute.

Turn-out & Storage:
Serve with whole grain baguette and shaved Romano cheese, over a cup of whole grain pasta, or alongside your favorite grilled or seared protein!

May be stored under refrigeration for up to 5 days.

**Not a part of traditional Ratatouille, but a great way to add protein to this dish!

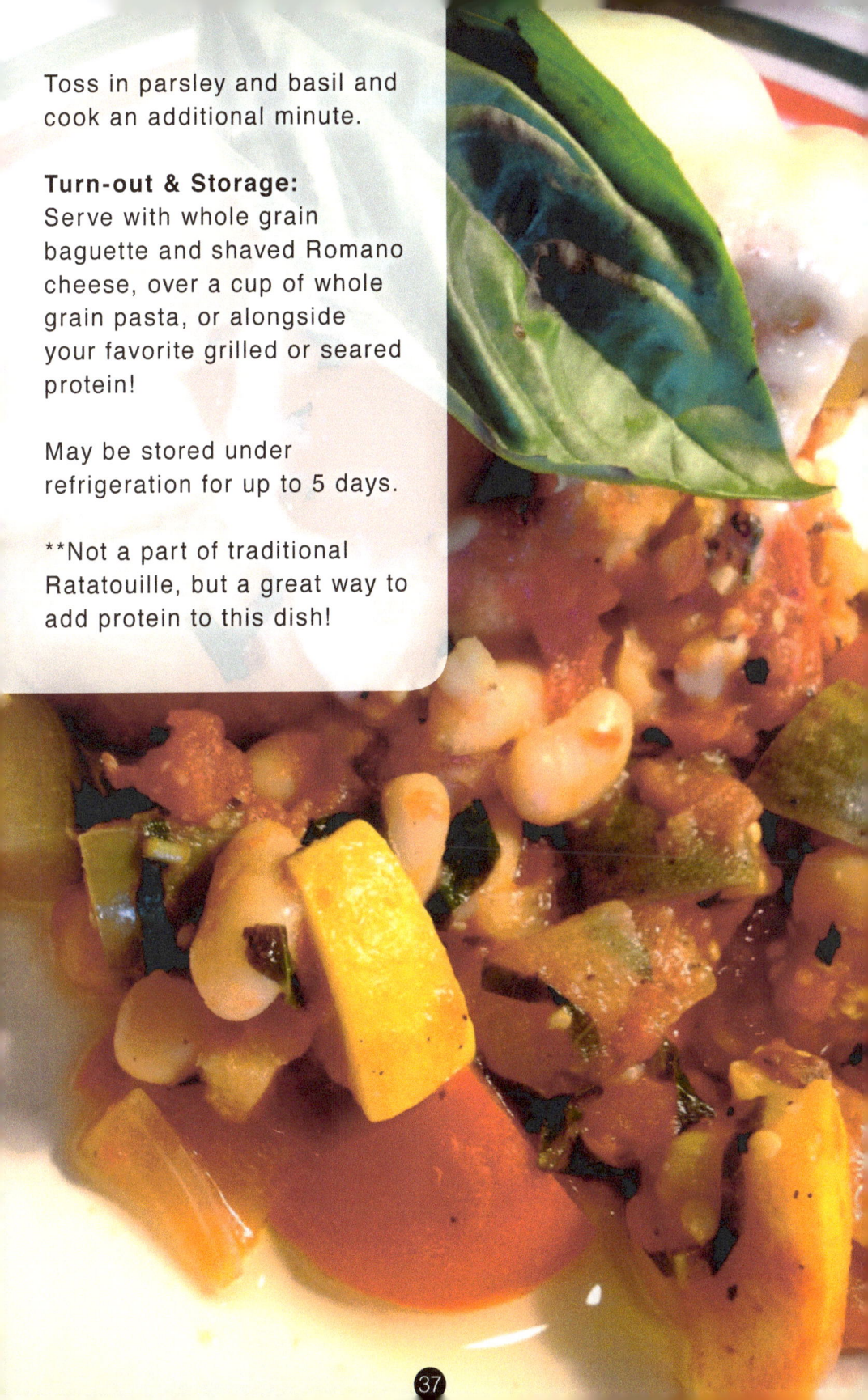

Mixed Berry Chai Quinoa Grits

ONE SERVING = 1 SLICE ON THE SLICE PLAN

Preparation Time: approximately 10 minutes
Cooking Time:　　　20 minutes
Serving Size:　　　½ cup mixture (Makes 6—8)

INGREDIENTS

2 cups .... water
1/2 tsp .... salt
4 TB .... chai powder mix
1 cup .... quinoa, washed for 30 minutes
1 cup .... berries, mixed (frozen/thawed or fresh):
　　　　　　　　　　blackberries, raspberries, blueberries, etc
1 tsp .... lemon juice
¼ cup .... raw sugar
½ cup .... milk
1 TB .... cornstarch

DIRECTIONS

Combine water and salt in saucepot; bring to a boil. Add chai and quinoa; stir. Cover, bring to a simmer (medium-low heat), and cook 15-20 minutes (depending on package instructions). Stir occasionally. Serve immediately.

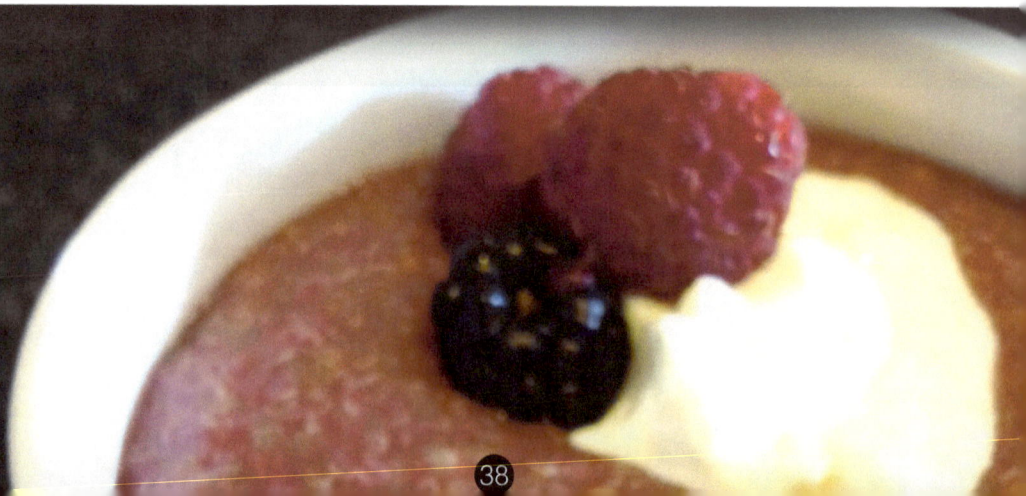

Beet, Potato, and Walnut Salad

ONE SERVING = 1 SLICE ON THE SLICE PLAN

Preparation Time: approximately 15 minutes
Cooking Time: about 45 minutes
Serving Size: 1 cup (Makes about 8)

INGREDIENTS

1 ½ lbs	beets, scrubbed, halved
1 ½ lbs	fingerling potatoes, halved lengthwise
3 TB	olive oil
3 TB	chervil, minced
2 TB	red wine vinegar
¼ cup	chives, fresh, chopped
½ cup	walnuts, chopped
1 TB	kosher salt (or to taste)
2 tsp.	black pepper (or to taste)

DIRECTIONS

Preheat oven to 450 degrees. Toss beets in 1 TB olive oil, seasoning with salt and pepper, and wrap in a large piece of aluminum foil forming a crimped pocket. Bake on wire rack for 30 minutes. Remove and allow to cool. Rub with a paper towel to remove outer skin (using gloves), and cut into ½"-1" cubes. Toss with vinegar and chives. Set aside.

Meanwhile, toss potatoes in remaining oil and season with salt and pepper. Arrange on baking dish, flesh side down. Bake 15 minutes. Toss potatoes and combine with walnuts. Cook until walnuts are toasted and potatoes are golden; about 8-10 minutes.

Turn-out & Storage:
Transfer potato walnut mixture to large bowl. Toss with beet mixture and chives; combine well. Serve immediately. Store for up to 3 days under refrigeration.

Pumpkin Spiced Smoothie

ONE SERVING = 2 SLICES ON THE SLICE PLAN

Preparation Time: approximately 5—7 minutes
Cooking Time: 15 minutes
Serving Size: 1 cup (Makes about 2)

INGREDIENTS

½ cup................. pumpkin puree
1 cup................. vanilla yogurt, fat free
1 .... apples, cored
1 .... banana, cut into pieces
1 TB................... honey
½ tsp................. vanilla extract
4 tsp. .... pumpkin pie spice
1 cup................. crushed ice

OPTIONAL GARNISH:
½ cup................. apples, cored and diced
½ cup................. granulated sugar
1/8 cup .... water
1/6 cup .... condensed skim milk

DIRECTIONS

Combine all ingredients in blender. Puree until smooth.

For garnish, combine sugar and water and cook until boiling. Stir with wooden spoon to combine and swirl (without stirring) until mixture becomes amber brown. Remove from heat and add milk. Stir in apples. Serve as garnish.

Turn-out & Storage: Store under refrigeration for no more than 3 days and serve cold.

Garnish with apple caramel topping, optional.

*Pumpkin is a squash high in beta-carotene, the precursor for vitamin A. Vitamin A plays an important role in the health of the cornea, epithelial cells, and mucus membranes; immune function as an antioxidant suppressing free radicals, bone health and maintenance, and assists in the regulation of gene expression by stimulation of gene transcription via retinoic acid.

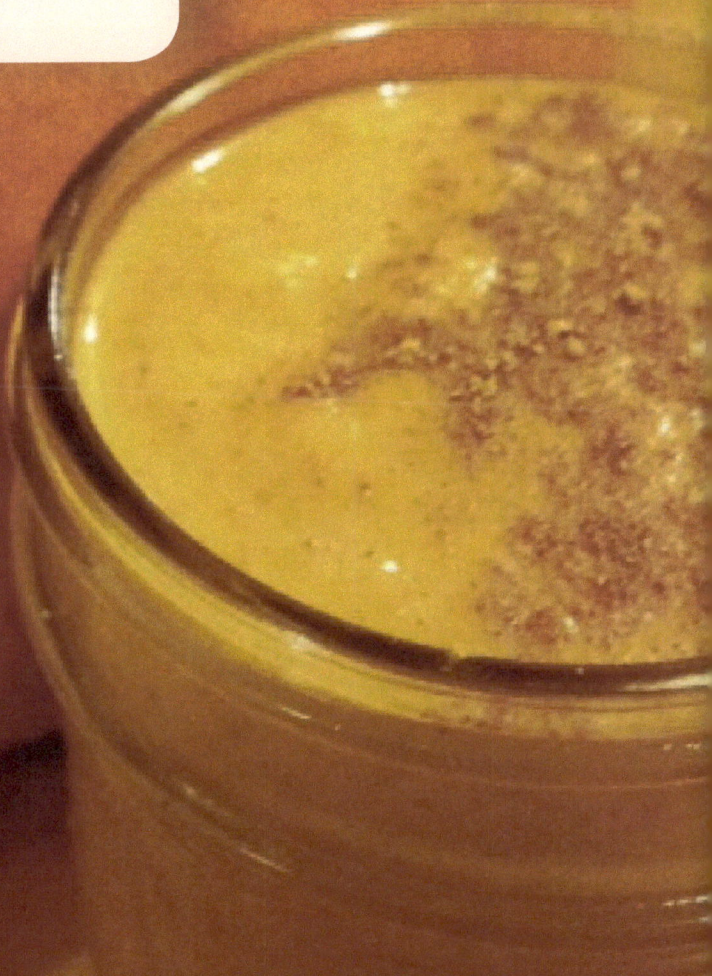

Grilled Pulled Chicken Sandwiches

ONE SERVING = 2 SLICES ON THE SLICE PLAN
(with a whole wheat roll)

Preparation Time: approximately 10 minutes
Cooking Time: 20—25 minutes
Serving Size: ½ cup mixture + 2 TB mushrooms
(Makes about 4)

INGREDIENTS

16 oz.................. chicken breast, boneless, skinless
2 tsp .... Worcestershire sauce
½ tsp.................. kosher salt
½ tsp.................. black pepper
¼ tsp.................. chili powder
½ tsp.................. garlic powder
½ lb. .... mushrooms, baby Portobello, sliced ¼" thick
1 TB................... olive oil
1 tsp .... garlic, fresh, chopped
2 cups................ arugula
2 oz .... goat cheese
4......................... whole grain rolls (or a roll of your choosing)

DIRECTIONS

Wash chicken breasts and pat dry. Rub both sides with Worcestershire sauce, salt, pepper, chili powder, and garlic powder. Place on grill and cook evenly on both sides until internal temperature of 155 degrees.

Meanwhile, heat olive oil in sauté pan. Add garlic and cook until slightly translucent. Add mushrooms and continue cooking until mushrooms are al dente. Set aside.

Prepare rolls by cutting in half and placing open-side down on grill. When slightly toasted, remove and spread with ½ oz goat cheese. Set aside. Remove chicken breasts from grill. Using two forks, pull chicken apart into large pieces (TIP: using tongs and a fork here may help as well if you are having trouble pulling apart the meat). Split into 4 equal sized portions.

Turn-out & Storage:

Place portioned chicken onto bottom of bun and top with mushroom mixture. Place ½ cup arugula on top and place the goat cheese covered top bun on to seal the sandwich.

Serve with grilled vegetables, polenta, or freshly cut melon.

Chicken and mushroom mixtures may be stored under refrigeration for up to 3 days.

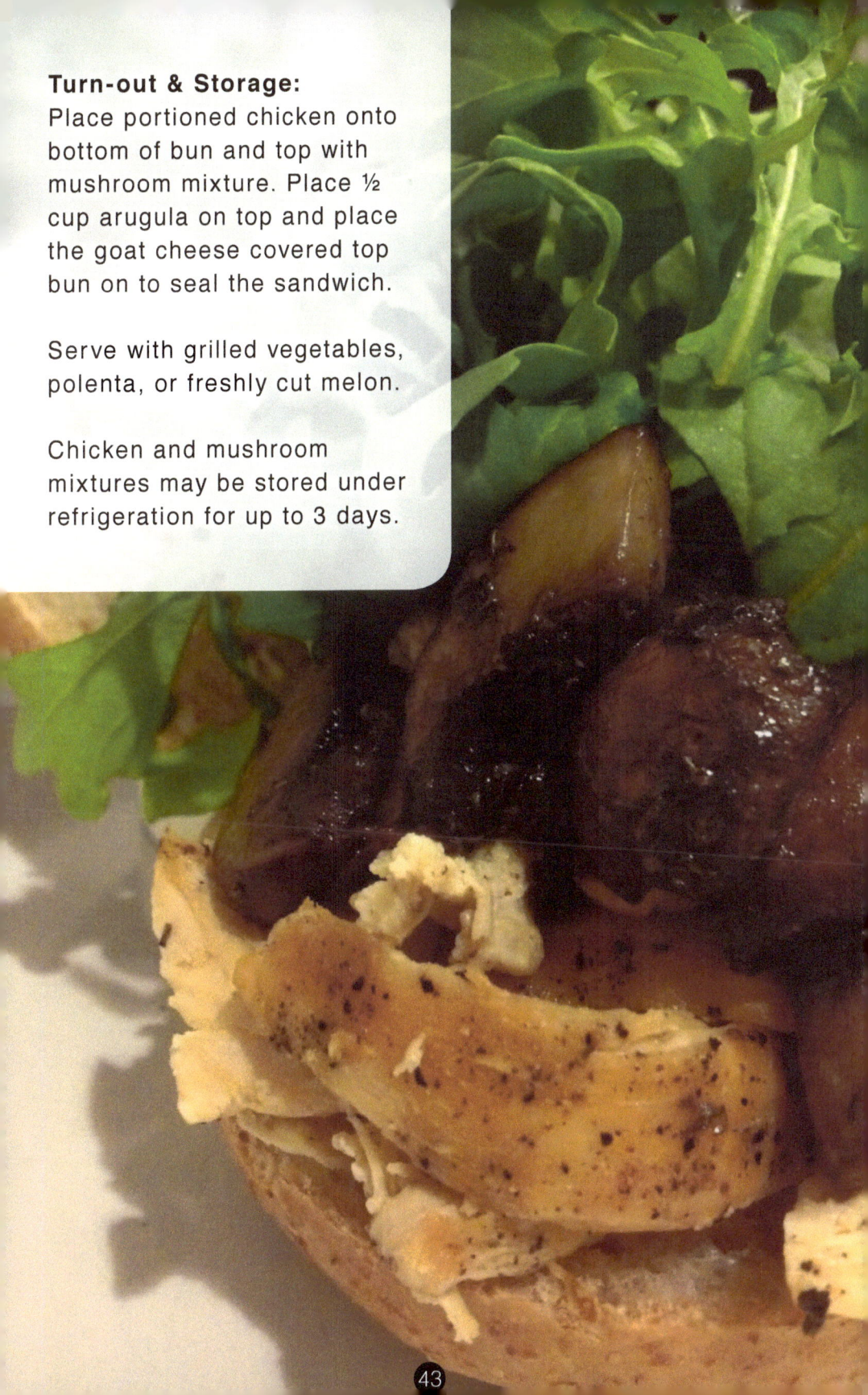

Spice Rubbed Grilled Lamb with Warm Mango Chutney

ONE SERVING = 0 SLICES ON THE SLICE PLAN

Preparation Time: approximately 15 minutes
Cooking Time: 6 minutes
Serving Size: 1 piece + ¼ cup chutney (Makes about 2)

INGREDIENTS

2........................ Lamb Loin Chops, 4 oz.

MANGO CHUTNEY

1........................ mango, diced
¼........................ pineapple, diced
1 larg................. shallot, minced
1/4 cup.............. lime juice
1 tsp.................. sugar (to taste)
1/8 tsp............... cayenne

SPICE BLEND

1/4 cup.............. olive oil
1 tsp.................. cumin
1 tsp.................. coriander
½ tsp................. chili powder
½ tsp................. cinnamon
1 tsp.................. black pepper
3/4 tsp.............. salt

DIRECTIONS

Toss together mango chutney ingredients in small bowl. In separate bowl, combine spice blend ingredients. Allow chutney to marinate at room temperature 20 minutes, tossing to combine occasionally.

Rub spice blend on lamb, both sides, until evenly coated. Meanwhile, heat grill, brush with oil, and sear both sides of lamb, creating an X before moving on to the alternate side. Cook lamb to desired doneness. Recommendation: medium. Toss chutney together before serving with lamb.

Turn-out & Storage:
Serve hot with salsa on side. Can substitute venison in recipe for lamb.

Chutney can be stored under refrigeration for up to 3 days.

Nutrition Note: Meats like lamb and venison are not only delicious as they have a different flavor compared to beef, chicken, or pork, but also are packed with nutrition. These meats have low marbling, which means they are leaner cuts of red meat. Also, these meats are high in protein, iron, choline, magnesium, and phosphorus.

Because iron is better absorbed with vitamin C, the ingredients in the chutney allow for better absorption of nutrients.

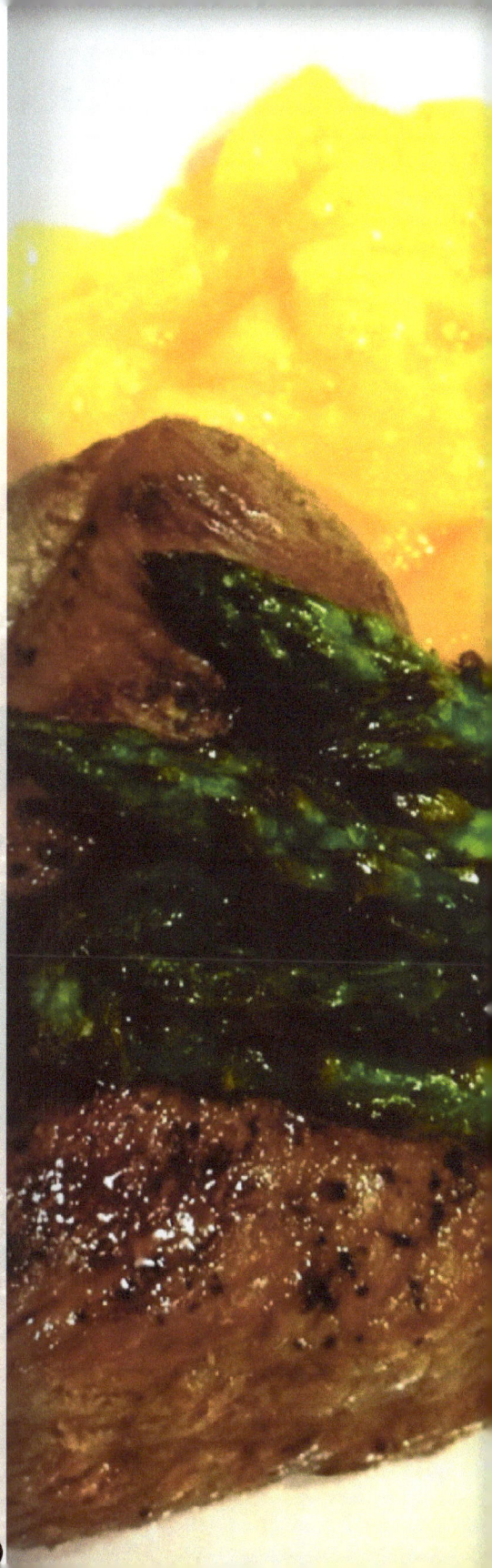

Asian Chicken Lettuce Wraps

ONE SERVING = 0 SLICES ON THE SLICE PLAN

Preparation Time: approximately 15 minutes
Cooking Time: 10—15 minutes
Serving Size: 1 wrap (Makes 4)

INGREDIENTS

4	leaves, Boston Bibb lettuce, washed
2	chicken breasts, diced into ½" cubes
1 TB	garlic, chopped
¼	green bell pepper, julienned
¼	red bell pepper, julienned
½ cup	yellow onion, small diced
½ cup	button mushrooms, sliced
1 TB	ginger, minced (or 2 tsp. dried ginger powder)
2 tsp	red pepper flakes
2 tsp	salt
2 TB	canola oil
1 TB	sesame oil
1 TB	soy sauce, low sodium
2 sprigs	cilantro, cleaned and dried
½ cup	almonds, sliced, toasted
¼ cup	peanut sauce, prepared

DIRECTIONS

Heat skillet with half the canola oil over medium heat. Sauté chicken, stirring often, until browned on all sides.

Add soy sauce, red pepper flakes, 1 tsp. salt and cook thoroughly until internal temperature of 150 degrees is reached.

Meanwhile, heat a second skillet with the other half of the canola oil over medium-high heat. Add onions and ginger and sauté until softened. Add bell peppers and mushrooms and cook until softer than al dente. Add 1 tsp. salt and sesame oil, tossing to coat thoroughly.

Turn-out & Storage:

Place open lettuce leaf and stuff with 1/4 chicken mixture. Top with 1/4 vegetable mixture and 1 TB peanut sauce.

Garnish with almonds and cilantro sprig. Enjoy!

Store almonds at room temperature whereas chicken and vegetable mixtures can be stored under refrigeration for no more than 3 days.

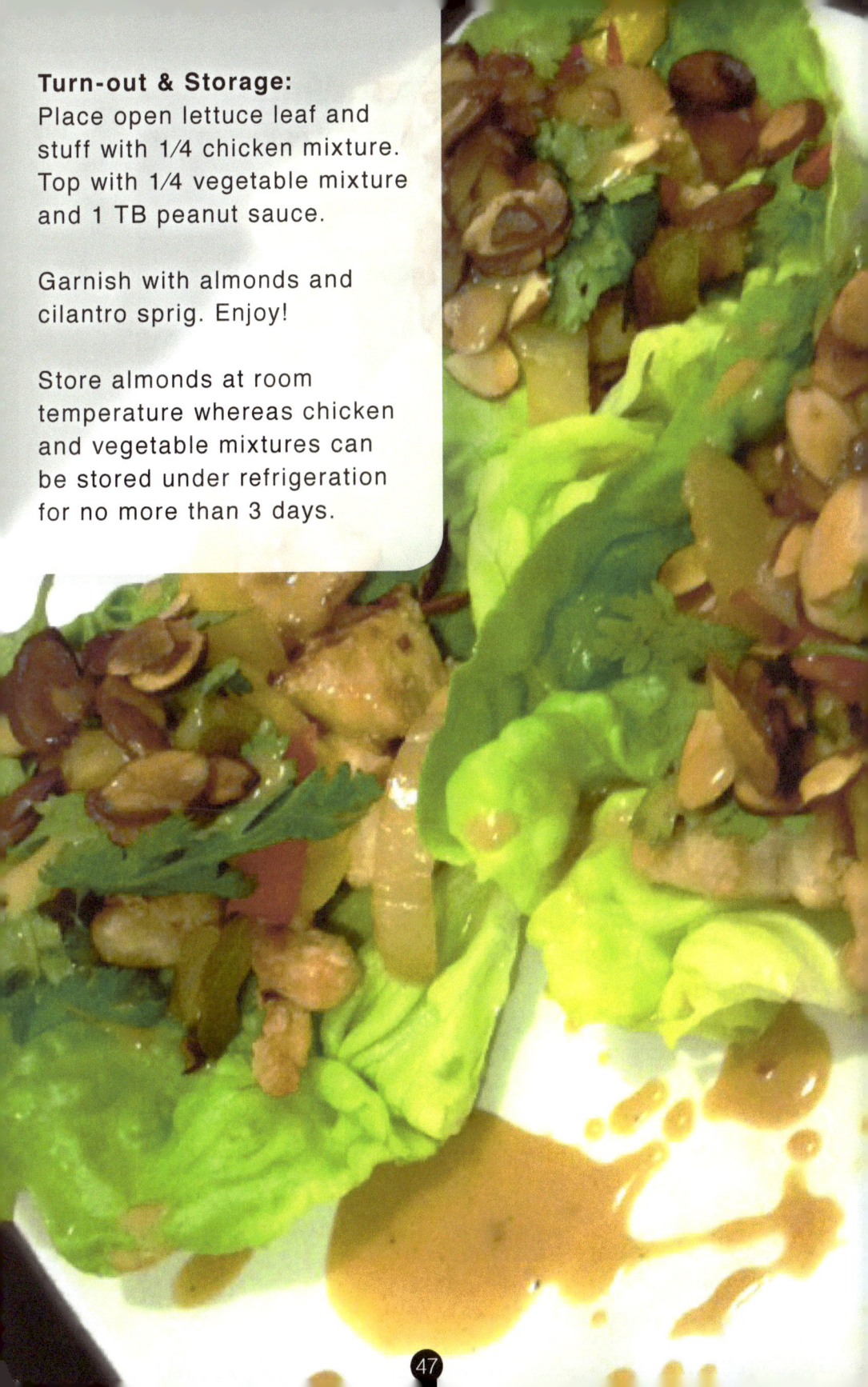

Honey Chipotle Roasted Wings

ONE SERVING = 0 SLICES ON THE SLICE PLAN

Preparation Time: approximately 5 minutes
Cooking Time: 1 minutes
Serving Size: 3 wings tossed in sauce (Makes about 18)

INGREDIENTS

3 lbs.................... chicken wings (approx. 18 wings)
3 TB .... baking powder
2 TB .... chili powder
1 TB .... kosher salt
2 cups................ orange juice
5 TB .... honey
1/4 cup .... soy sauce
2 tsp .... cornstarch
2 tsp .... chipotle chiles in adobo sauce, minced
1 TB .... ketchup
1 tsp .... cayenne pepper
garnish............... cilantro

DIRECTIONS

Heat oven to 400 degrees. Rinse wings well and dab with a paper towel to dry. Meanwhile, blend baking powder, chili powder, and salt. Toss wings in mixture to lightly coat. Place on baking rack on top of baking pan; Roast 30 minutes.

Meanwhile, prepare the sauce by combining the orange juice, honey, soy sauce, chipotles/ adobo, and cayenne into a saucepan over medium heat. Simmer 5-8 minutes until slightly thickened. Create a slurry by removing 2 TB liquid and mixing with cornstarch – add back to mixture and allow to thicken the rest of the way.

After 30 minutes have passed, remove the wings from the oven and coat with the glaze thoroughly. You can place them into a bowl, toss with the sauce, and replace them on the rack, if desired. Bake for an additional 15 minutes.

Turn-out & Storage:
Serve immediately; garnish with cilantro.

Sauce may be stored under refrigeration for up to 7 days.

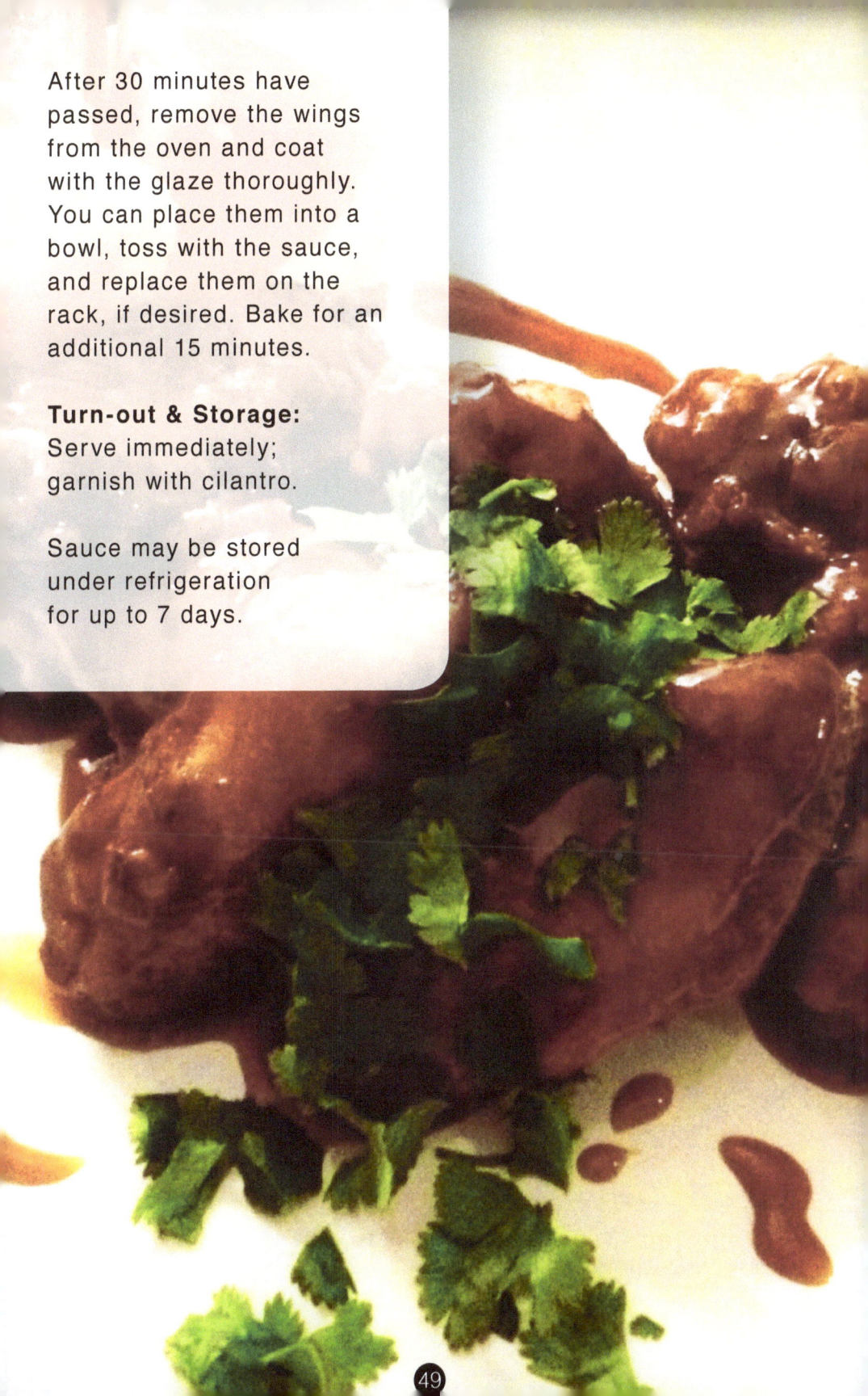

Halibut with Strawberry Salsa

ONE SERVING = 0 SLICES ON THE SLICE PLAN

Preparation Time: approximately 15 minutes
Cooking Time: 6 minutes
Serving Size: 1 piece + ½ cup salsa (Makes 2)

INGREDIENTS

1 pint .... strawberries- fresh, washed, stemmed, and diced
1 TB.................... red onion, diced small
1........................ scallion, chopped fine
1 small .... garlic clove, minced
1 small .... jalapeño, sliced into thin rings
1........................ lime, juice of
1 TB.................... orange juice
1 TB.................... cilantro, minced
2- 6 oz .... halibut filets, skin on
To Taste .... kosher salt and black pepper
As needed .... olive oil

DIRECTIONS

Toss together strawberries, onion, scallion, garlic, jalapeño, lime juice, orange juice, and cilantro. Allow to marinate at room temperature 20-30 minutes (overnight OK too). Toss again and adjust seasonings, if necessary.

Season each side of halibut with salt and pepper. Heat 1-2 TB olive oil in sauté pan and sear halibut, skin side down first, until crispy and color rises half up the outside of filet. Turn and sear opposite side until all sides change color and fish feels somewhat firm to the touch. This fish can be served medium.

Toss salsa together before serving with fish.

Turn-out & Storage: Serve hot with salsa on side.

Can substitute for any thick cut fish filet, such as salmon.

Salsa can be stored under refrigeration for up to 3 days.

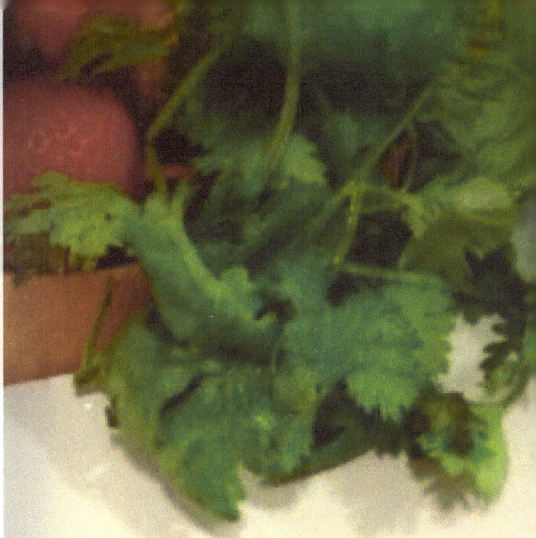

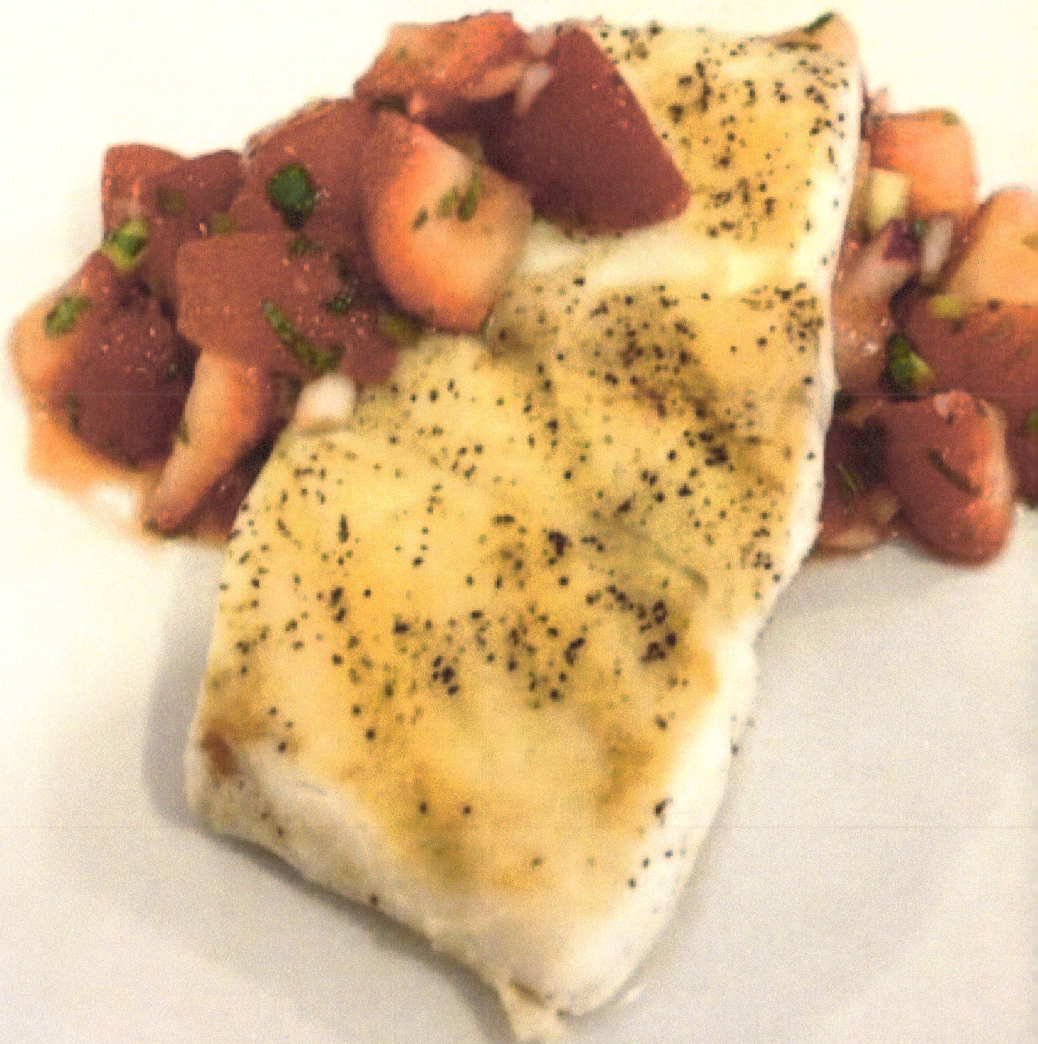

Garden Fresh Lasagna

ONE SERVING = 0 SLICES ON THE SLICE PLAN

Preparation Time: approximately 20 minutes
Cooking Time: 45 minutes — 1 hour
Serving Size: 1 - 3x3" square (Makes 12)

<u>INGREDIENTS</u>

4	zucchini (medium), sliced lengthwise
2	eggplant (large), peeled and sliced lengthwise
1 bunch	kale, blanched and de-stemmed
2 tsp	nutmeg*
6 oz	mozzarella cheese (skim/part-skim), shredded

VEGGIE MIXTURE

2 TB	olive oil
1	onion (medium), diced
1 TB	garlic, minced
1 cup	carrot, diced
8 oz	mushrooms (button), diced
1	green bell pepper, diced
1	red bell pepper, diced
1-28 oz can	whole tomatoes, no salt added (with juice)
1 TB	oregano, dried (or 2 TB freshly chopped)
1 TB	rosemary, dried (or 2 TB freshly chopped)
2 TB	tomato paste, no salt added
¼ cup	red wine
¼ cup	parsley, chopped
¼ cup	basil, chopped
½ tsp	red pepper flakes
2 tsp	salt
1 tsp	sugar granules, raw**

CHEESE MIXTURE

24 oz	ricotta cheese, skim/part-skim
½ cup	grated Parmesan cheese
12 oz	mozzarella cheese (skim/part-skim), shredded
1	egg, beaten
2 tsp	black pepper
1 TB	oregano, dried (you may also use dried Italian Seasoning)

DIRECTIONS

Preheat oven to 350 degrees. Grease a 9x13" baking pan with cooking spray or dabbing a paper towel with olive oil.

Combine ingredients for cheese mixture and set aside under refrigeration. Meanwhile, begin preparing the vegetable mixture by heating a skillet with olive oil. Add onion and garlic; sauté until translucent. Add carrots and heat until slightly harder than al dente. Add bell peppers and mushrooms and continue cooking 5 minutes. Deglaze pan with red wine. Add whole tomatoes, breaking them up with your hands as they are added. Stir in tomato paste, parsley, herbs, red pepper flakes, salt, and sugar. Mix well. Set aside.

Place ½ cup sauce/vegetable mixture on bottom of baking pan. Layer with eggplant and zucchini on one even layer, topping with one layer of kale (that is tossed with nutmeg). Top half of the cheese mixture followed by another layer of eggplant, zucchini, and kale, as previously directed. Follow with another layer of the remaining sauce/ vegetable mixture then the remainder of the cheese mixture. Top with a last layer of eggplant, zucchini, and kale followed by the last third of sauce/vegetable mixture. Bake for 30 minutes, covered (with foil), until internal temperature of 145 degrees is reached. Uncover, top with 6 oz mozzarella, and continue baking for 15 minutes until cheese is melted and somewhat browned. Remove from heat and allow to set 10 minutes.

Turn-out & Storage:
Serve 3x3 square; garnish with parmesan cheese or basil leaves. Accompany with whole grain pasta tossed in olive oil (optional). Can be stored under refrigeration for up to 3 days.

*Nutmeg should always accompany dark leafy greens, such as kale, in order to enhance flavor and add health benefits.
**A little sugar should be added to tomato products (especially canned) to offset the acidity.

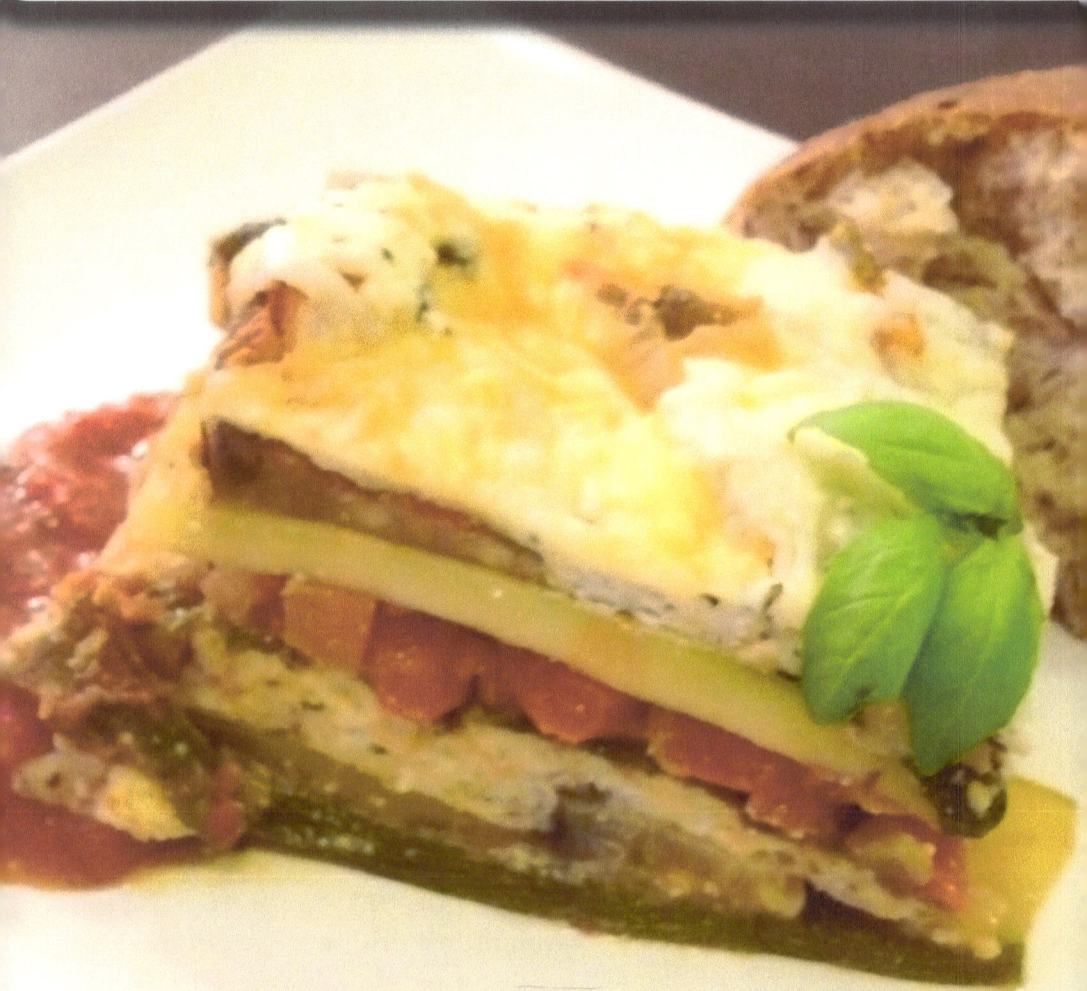

Spicy Apple Salsa

ONE SERVING = 0 SLICES ON THE SLICE PLAN

Preparation Time: approximately 10 minutes
Cooking Time: N/a
Serving Size: 1 - 3x3" square (Makes 12)

INGREDIENTS

3 .... green apples, small diced
½ .... red onion, diced small
1 .... jalepeño, chopped fine
1 .... lime, juice and zest of
¼ cup .... cilantro, minced
2 tsp .... garlic, minced
2 tsp .... oregano, fresh, minced
1-2 tsp. .... granulated sugar (optional)
2 TB................... olive oil
To Taste .... kosher salt

DIRECTIONS

Combine ingredients in large
bowl and mix well.

Turn-out & Storage:
Rest under refrigeration,
covered, 2 hours or more.
Store chilled and serve cold.

May be stored under
refrigeration for up to 3 days.

Chickpea Chole

ONE SERVING = 1.5 SLICES ON THE SLICE PLAN
(with 1/3 cup of rice)

Preparation Time: approximately 15 minutes
Cooking Time: 25—30 minutes
Serving Size: ¾ cup mixture (Makes about 6)

INGREDIENTS

2 TB................... olive oil
1 TB................... garlic
1...................... onion, yellow, large
1...................... green bell pepper
2 tsp .... cumin
1 tsp .... coriander powder
1 tsp .... turmeric
1 tsp .... ginger powder
2 tsp .... fennel seed
2 tsp .... chili powder
2 tsp .... curry powder
2- 15.5 oz .... fire-roasted diced tomatoes, canned, no-salt added
1- 15.5 oz .... garbanzo beans (chickpeas), canned, no-salt added
3 oz .... plain nonfat Greek Yogurt
2 TB................... cilantro, chopped roughly
Garnish .... almonds, slivered

DIRECTIONS

Heat olive oil in pot with a large base. Sauté garlic and onion about 2 minutes over medium-high heat, or until slightly softened. Add green bell pepper and continue cooking over medium heat, until peppers are softened. Onions and garlic should be translucent at this point.

Return to medium-high heat, add additional olive oil (if mixture has become dry), and add spices: cumin, coriander, turmeric, ginger, fennel seed, chili powder, and curry powder. Continue stirring (do not stop) until the oils of the spices are released and become aromatic.

Add diced tomatoes, return to medium/medium-low heat, and cover. Allow to simmer for 10 minutes, stirring occasionally. Remove cover and add chickpeas; cover again and cook for an additional 10 minutes, stirring occasionally.

Add Greek Yogurt and cilantro, stirring to combine.

Turn-out & Storage:
Serve immediately; garnish with slivered almonds. Great over brown rice, quinoa, or served with whole wheat pita wedges.

May be stored under refrigeration for up to 3 days.

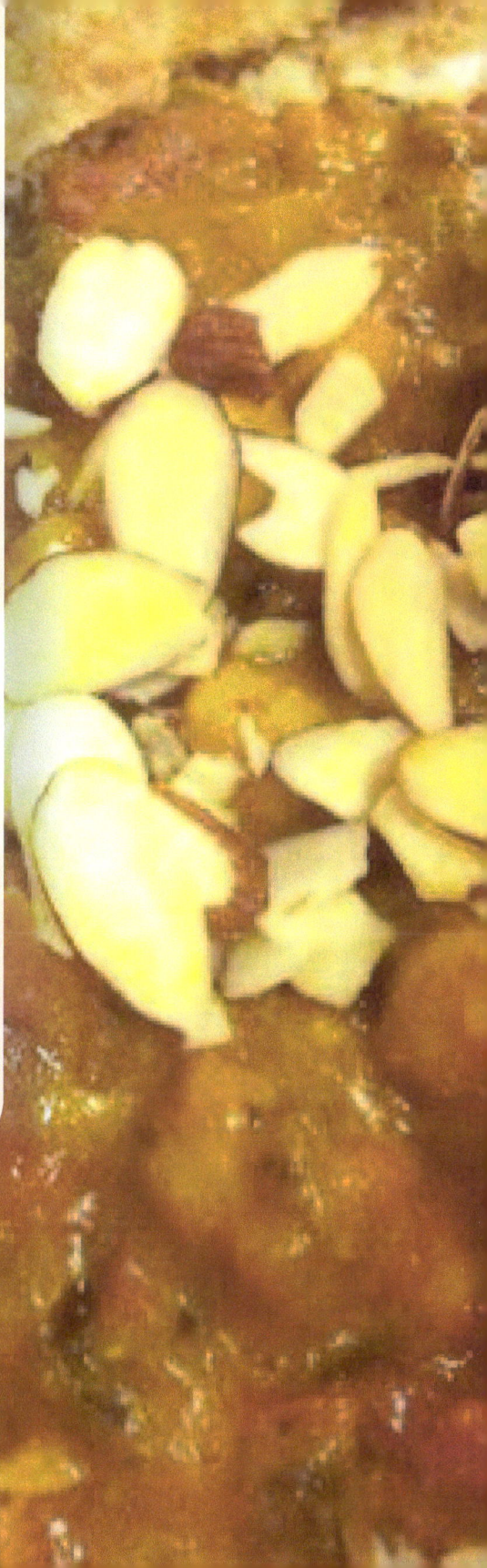

Butter Poached Eggs with Sorrel Pesto over Toast Points

ONE SERVING = 1 SLICE ON THE SLICE PLAN

Preparation Time: approximately 10 minutes
Cooking Time: 20 minutes
Serving Size: 1 piece

INGREDIENTS

6....................... eggs
1- 6"................... Italian bread loaf, sliced on bias into ½- ¾ inch pieces
garnish.............. scallions, chopped

SORREL PESTO
1 bunch.............. sorrel leaves, about 2 packed cups
2 cloves............. garlic
1/4 cup .... walnuts
1/4 cup .... fresh parmesan cheese
1/4 cup .... extra virgin olive oil
To Taste .... Salt and pepper

BUERRE NANTAIS
1/2 cup .... unsalted butter
2 TB .... dry white wine
2 TB.................. white-wine vinegar
1 TB .... chopped shallot
3 TB .... heavy cream
¼ tsp .... fresh lemon juice

DIRECTIONS

To prepare pesto: Combine garlic, walnuts, and parmesan cheese in food processor and pulse until the mixture has a coarse texture. Add in sorrel leaves and pulse until combined. Stream in olive oil until nappe. Season with salt and pepper. Set aside.

To prepare buerre nantais:
Cut butter into small
pieces and chill. In a small
heavy saucepan simmer
wine, vinegar, and shallot
over moderate heat until
liquid is reduced to about
1 tablespoon, about 5
minutes. Add cream and
simmer mixture until slightly
thickened, about 2 minutes.
Gradually add butter a few
pieces at a time, whisking
and adding more before
previous pieces are fully
incorporated (mixture
will be creamy and pale).
Season sauce with lemon
juice and salt and pepper.

Break eggs directly into sauce
and cover, reducing heat to
a simmer. Cook until whites
are fully cooked (yolks will
be soft). Meanwhile, drizzle
slices of bread with olive oil
and toast until golden brown.

Turn-out & Storage: Spread
about 1 TB sorrel pesto
over toast point. Top with
poached egg (without sauce),
and garnish with scallions.
Sauce is optional and should
be disposed after cooking
with eggs. Serve this dish
with freshly cut fruit, roasted
asparagus, or freshly cut
tomatoes topped with goat
cheese and black pepper.

Autumn Quinoa Salad

ONE SERVING = 1 SLICE ON THE SLICE PLAN

Preparation Time: approximately 10 minutes
Cooking Time: 12—15 minutes
Serving Size: 1 cup (Makes about 3)

INGREDIENTS

SALAD

¾ cup................. Quinoa, rinsed and dried
1 ½ cups .... water
4 oz. .... kale, blanched and cooled
3 TB.................. pumpkin seeds, no shell
¼ cup................ dried cranberries
¾ cup................ apples, small diced
2 tsp. .... salt
1 tsp. .... nutmeg*

DRESSING

4 TB.................. Apple cider
3 TB.................. White vinegar
9 TB.................. Olive oil
1 tsp. .... Dijon mustard
2 tsp .... Kosher salt
1 tsp .... White pepper

DIRECTIONS

Add water, salt, and quinoa to pot and heat over medium heat until boiling. Cover and simmer 12-15 minutes or until water has completely dissolved and outer shell of quinoa is broken. Cool.

Meanwhile, combine kale and nutmeg. Toss with remaining salad ingredients together with quinoa mixture.

To prepare the dressing: add vinegar, salt, and pepper to bowl. Slowly drizzle oil whisking continuously to combine. Add mustard to emulsify. Add apple cider. Toss with salad and allow to stand at least 1 hour before serving.

Turn-out & Storage:
Serve chilled or at room temperature.

Store under refrigeration for no more than 3 days and serve cold or at room temperature.

*Nutmeg is an antioxidant that contains Trolox, a water-soluble form of vitamin E. Vitamin E is useful in protecting polyunsaturated fats (allowing them to get digested), supporting immunity, quenching free radicals, and supports normal nerve development. It also helps balance the harsh flavor of kale and release some of the natural flavors using very little.

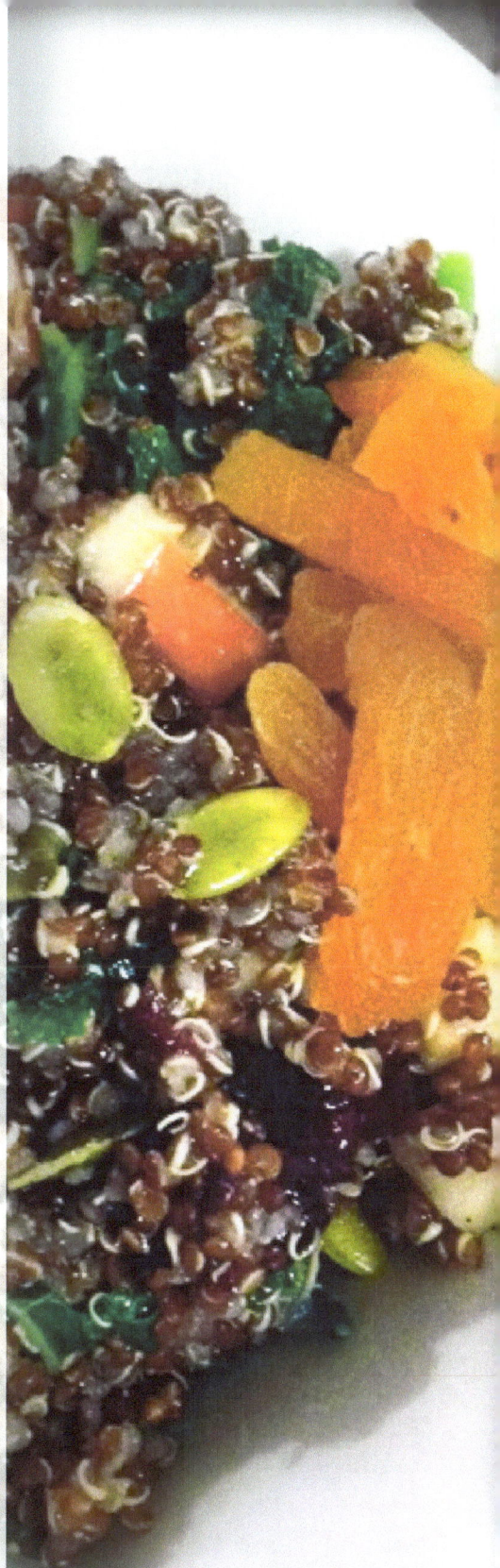

Beet Risotto

Preparation Time: approximately 45 — 60 minutes
Cooking Time: 30—35 minutes
Serving Size: ½ cup (Makes about 6)

INGREDIENTS

BEETS
1 TB.................... olive oil
2...................... beets, washed and halved

RISOTTO
1 TB.................... olive oil
1 .... red onion, small, diced
½ cup................. white wine
2 tsp .... thyme leaves, minced
1 cup.................. Arborio rice
3 cups............... chicken stock, reduced sodium
2 TB.................... butter
¼ cup................. Parmesan cheese, grated
To Taste .... salt and pepper

DIRECTIONS

Preheat oven to 400 degrees. Toss beets in oil and wrap in aluminum foil. Place in oven for 45 minutes-1 hour until soft. Remove from oven and quickly peel skin off. Set aside to cool. Cube into ½ inch pieces.

Meanwhile, heat stock on medium to simmering and reduce to low. Keep warm.

Heat olive oil in skillet and sauté onion until translucent. Add rice and toss to coat. Add white wine to deglaze pan. Stir in 1 cup stock and thyme. Simmer and stir occasionally. When liquid reduces by a half, add another cup of stock. Repeat until all stock is gone.

When final liquid is reduced by half, add cubed beets and stir. Add parmesan cheese and allow to cook until most risotto thickens to a creamy consistency. Stir in butter; season with salt/pepper.

Turn-out & Storage:
Serve alongside seared lamb, roasted pork, or grilled vegetables. Also good as an entrée in 1 cup portions.

Allow to cool before storing – will keep for up to three days under refrigeration.

Collard Greens

ONE SERVING = 0 SLICES ON THE SLICE PLAN

Preparation Time: approximately 10 minutes
Cooking Time: approximately 2 hours
Serving Size: ½ cup

INGREDIENTS

2 TB..................... olive oil
½ lb. .... smoked turkey breast, cut into small cubes
½ .... yellow onion, medium
2 TB..................... garlic, rough chopped
1 large bunch ..... collard greens
4 cups .... water + 2 TB salt (or reduced
                      sodium chicken stock)
2 TB .... granulated sugar
1 tsp .... crushed red pepper flakes
½ .... lemon, juice of
½ tsp................. nutmeg, ground

DIRECTIONS

In a pot, sauté turkey breast, onion, and garlic until turkey is browned and onion/garlic are translucent. Add liquid (water or stock) and bring to a boil. Cover, reduce heat to medium, and simmer for 20 minutes.

MEANWHILE, Break apart the collards: remove the stems that run down the center by holding the leaf in your left hand and stripping the leaf down with your right hand. You do not need to do this step to the young, tender leaves. Slice the greens by stacking on top of one another, rolling them up, and slicing in 1" thick pieces.

Place greens in pot; add remaining ingredients.

TIP #1: Wash the collard greens thoroughly. This will ensure no sand gets in your mouth!

TIP #2: Lemon juice and nutmeg may sound weird here, but they should not be tasted. The citrus in the lemon will bring out iron from the greens, while nutmeg overall enhances the flavor the greens have.

Cook for 45 to 60 minutes, stirring occasionally. Taste and adjust seasoning.

Turn-out & Storage:
Serve hot.

This can be stored for up to 3 days under refrigeration.

This is a unique and healthy twist of an original. Browning the turkey with the enhancement of onion and garlic flavors give this traditional American dish a well rounded taste. Collard greens are a healthy green rich in iron, but it must be released with vitamin C (hence the use of lemon juice). Serve with grilled chicken breast or alone with whole grain crusty bread.

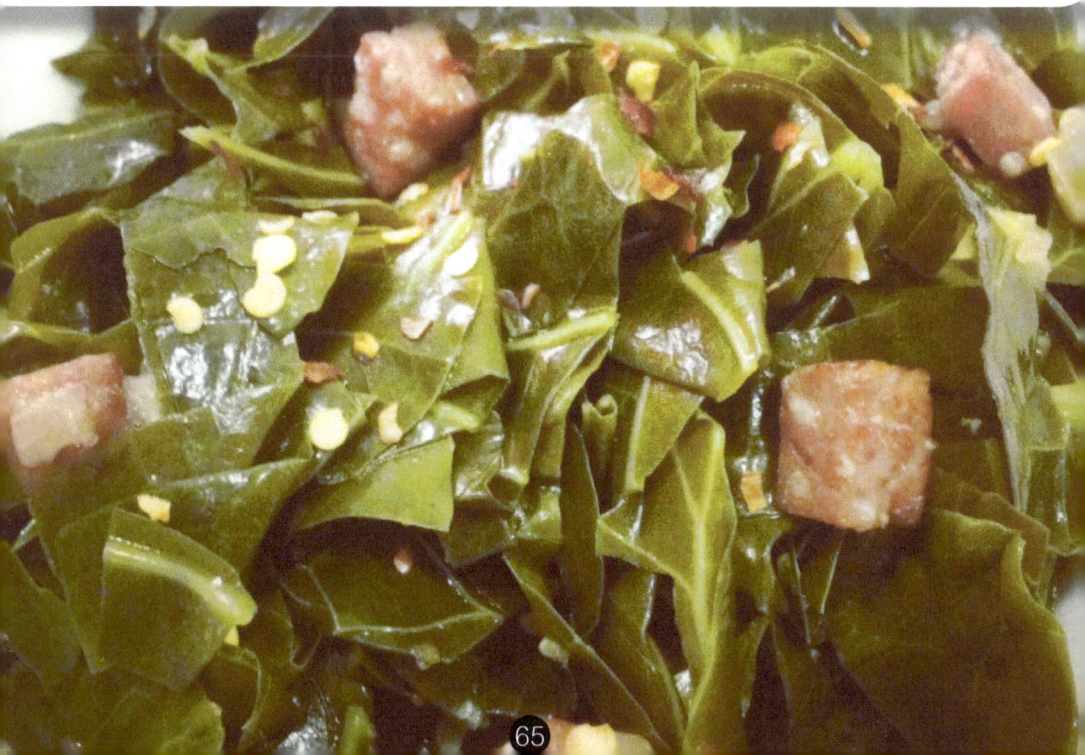

Conclusion

Using the Plan

Carbohydrates are important and should not be ignored. Notice that the Slice Plan focuses primarily on starchy foods and carbohydrates. However, using the MyPlate image as a guide for meals is necessary for the plan to work. Remember, your plate should be mostly fruits and vegetables. In a lot of the recipes throughout this book, there are uses of lean meats, low fat dairy, healthy protein and fats. The flavors within these recipes do not require additional salt. This serves to support which Foods to Choose Less and which Foods to Choose More.

Though Slices are the main component of this Plan, they are not the only element. Healthier options (including snacks), smaller portions, and physical activity are all vital for the Plan to work for you. If a recipe has Zero Slices, this does not mean you can eat unlimited amounts of these foods. Simply, it means that these items do not add Slices and are part of a healthy meal for that day. In its entirety, the Slice Plan integrates the benefits of living to enjoy your food with a calorie-cutting regimen and support from someone who cares.

If you follow this plan for lifestyle change, it WILL work... whether your goal is weight loss, reduced cholesterol, lowered blood pressure, or you just want to live a healthier life. Remember healthy weight loss is about 1-2 pounds per week, the rest is reward! Sometimes, starting a new dietary lifestyle means losing more weight in the beginning and reaching a plateau later on. This is common, and not something to discourage you.

This plan incorporates all of the aspects of healthy living:

✔ Reduced caloric intake

✔ Moderate carbohydrate intake

✔ Low fat and salt

✔ Incorporation of healthy fats and whole grains

✔ Plenty of fruits and vegetables

✔ Avoidance of unhealthy diet practices

✔ Keeping the foods you love part of your life!

The only missing component is physical activity. So GET MOVING! Do what you love to do and do not feel like a "slave to the gym." Aim for a total of 150 minutes per week.

• Walk, Run, or Jog outdoors

• Yoga or Pilates

• Biking outdoors or Cycling indoors

• Play your favorite sport: basketball, volleyball, soccer, tennis

• Join the gym – consider a personal trainer

This Plan is unique because you have a registered dietitian and professional chef on your side to provide one on one counseling, assistance + guidance, recipe suggestions, and reinforcement while you are getting started or feel in a rut.

Thank you for your trust, time and effort...
and remember, you *can* do this!

Contact Zachari Breeding, RD
thesageculinary@gmail.com
facebook.com/mrcookit
the-sage.org